101 Dog Tricks

QUARRY

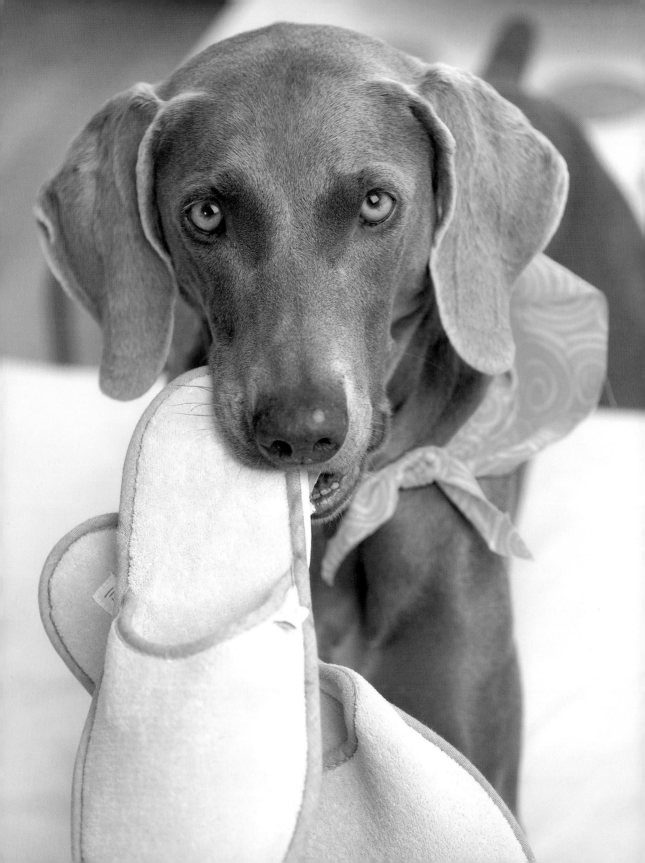

101 Dog Tricks

Step-by-Step Activities to Engage, Challenge, and Bond with Your Dog

Kyra Sundance and Chalcy

Photography by Nick Saglimbeni

BEVERLY MASSACHUSETTS

QUARRY BOOKS

First published in the United States of America by
Quarry Books, a member of
Quarto Publishing Group USA Inc.
100 Cummings Center, Suite 406-L
Beverly, Massachusetts 01915
Telephone: (978) 282-3575
Fax: (978) 282-7765

Library of Congress Cataloging-in-Publication Data available

ISBN-13: 978-1-59253-325-1
ISBN-10: 1-59253-325-6

17 16 15   41

101 Dog Tricks contains a variety of training recommendations for your dog. While caution was taken to give safe recommendations, it is impossible to predict an individual dog's reaction to the recommended handling or training. Neither the author, Kyra Sundance, Sundance MediaCom, nor the Publisher, Quarto Publishing Group USA Inc., accepts liability for any mental, financial, or physical harm that arises from following the advice, techniques, or procedures in this book. Readers should use personal judgment when applying the recommendations of this text.

Cover Design: Rockport Publishers
Design: Sundance MediaCom
www.sundancemediacom.com
All photography: Nick Saglimbeni/www.slickforce.com, with the exception of the following: Kyra Sundance, 10, 11, 12, 13, 20, 21, 34, 50, 84, 104, 106, 142, 159, 178, and 208.
"Do More With Your Dog!" is a registered trademark of Kyra Sundance.

Printed in China

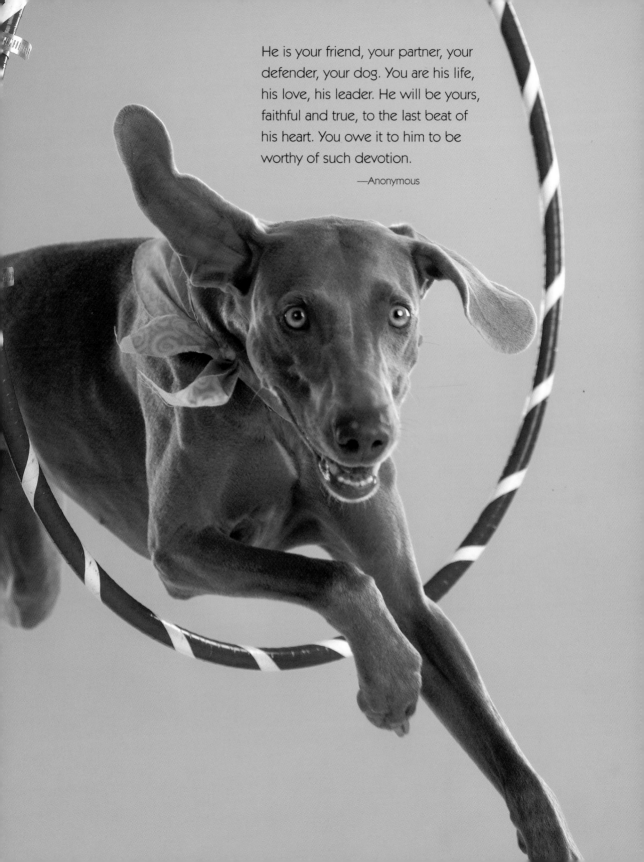

He is your friend, your partner, your defender, your dog. You are his life, his love, his leader. He will be yours, faithful and true, to the last beat of his heart. You owe it to him to be worthy of such devotion.

—Anonymous

CONTENTS

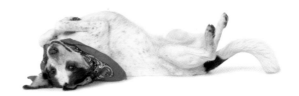

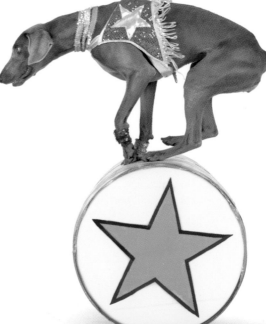

FOREWORD

By Bill Langworthy

I first met Kyra and Chalcy while I was producing an animal talent show for television. One of the bookers announced she had found a dog who could read! In all my years of working with pet tricks, first as David Letterman's Stupid Pet Tricks Coordinator then as a producer on Animal Planet's *Pet Star,* I'd heard of some clever animals, but I had a feeling this one was special. Sure enough, Kyra and Chalcy promptly won the show, then came back and won in the championships!

Two things about Kyra and Chalcy stand out in my memory: first, their big smiles; and second, they did everything together. The camera can make people focus on themselves, forgetting they're only half of a team, but from the first rehearsal to the final championship round, Kyra and Chalcy did everything together. When Kyra phoned me and said, "Chalcy and I are writing a book," I wasn't surprised—my only question was, "Who typed?"

101 Dog Tricks is all about doing things as a team. Kyra and Chalcy use only positive training and motivational techniques to reinforce trick training as a fun way to play rather than a chore. The tricks are all designed to develop a particular aspect of your dog's abilities, from the mental to the physical, while also developing trust and friendship between you and your companion.

Kyra and Chalcy know every trick in the book; that is, they have practiced and performed all 101 routines, so *101 Dog Tricks* is filled with firsthand advice. Kyra and Chalcy are equally adept in both mental and physical tricks, so you'll find instruction on everything from teaching your dog to count to teaching your dog to play basketball. The instructions are clearly illustrated and easy to follow, but no detail has been spared. This is the one and only book every trick trainer needs, whether you plan to entertain yourself, your friends, or huge crowds and national television audiences like Kyra and Chalcy.

Kyra Sundance and Chalcy are uniquely qualified to write the definitive trick training book. It's every trick trainer's privilege that Kyra and Chalcy took time from their performing schedule to share their secrets. So enjoy this book, then get outside and play. As Kyra and Chalcy always say: "Do More With Your Dog!®"

Bill Langworthy spent many years as a pet trick coordinator for Late Show with David Letterman *and a writer and coproducer of* Animal Planet's *"Pet Star" talent competition. He's auditioned thousands of animal acts across the country.*

AUTHORS' NOTE

"See?" I said, "Chalcy keeps missing the weave pole entrance."

"You should have taught her initially using the two-pole method" advised the nationally ranked agility coach. "Dogs who start with the two-pole method never miss an entrance."

"Well, we didn't." I admitted, "We trained a different method. So this is where we're at now. How do we fix it?" I asked. She shook her head.

"Oh, it's too late now," said the coach as she walked off.

This coach was of the opinion that since I'd screwed up my dog by using the wrong training method, I should cut my losses and make a fresh start with a new agility dog. In other words, don't waste your time fixing something when you can buy a newer, shinier one for cheaper!

Needless to say, I didn't give up on Chalcy. I can't begin to list all the training mistakes I've made with her over the years. I've taught her wrong things, using wrong methods, while giving wrong feedback. Sure, I'd messed up in our training, but we fixed it! We went back and retaught skills and relearned rules. It's a little harder this way, granted, but certainly possible. I don't expect my dog to be a machine, and I'm not one either. We try, we learn, we fail, we succeed. We work together and afford each other endless second chances. We still miss the occasional weave pole entrance, but we never miss the opportunity to give it one more go!

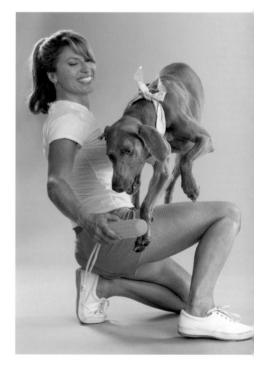

Whether your dog is young or old, athletic or lazy, quick-witted or dumb as a rock, he's *your* dog and his success need only be measured in *your* eyes.

I hope this book inspires you to not only teach tricks, but to "Do More With Your Dog!®"

—Kyra Sundance and Chalcy

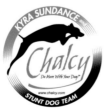

Rover knows when you are preparing for a trip. Fido hears the word "bath" or "vet" and takes cover under the bed. Spot senses when you've had a bad day and lays his head in your lap, and Buster nudges your arm as you sit on the couch trying to find the motivation to go for a walk. These examples of human/dog communication illustrate the familial relationship dogs play in our lives. And this relationship, as with any positive relationship in our lives, requires nurturing to keep it alive and flourishing.

Trick training is a way to build upon this relationship, establishing communication methods, trust, and mutual respect. It offers a way to bond with your dog as you strive toward common goals and delight in your successes. It deepens paths of communication, built through repetition and effort.

If you've ever tried to communicate a message to a person who speaks a foreign language, you've probably tried a combination of pantomime, pictographs, sound mimicry, and other tactics quite hilarious to onlookers. But when that message finally gets communicated... "Ahhh! The goat cheese pizza!"... there is a feeling of mutual success and bonding. That same joy and bond can be achieved by you and your dog as you work together on dog tricks!

Trick training does more than teach cute party tricks to entertain your friends. Trick training offers an opportunity to better understand how your dog thinks and have him better understand your cues. The trust and cooperative spirit developed through this process will last a lifetime.

HOW TO USE THIS BOOK

Start anywhere! Each trick displays a difficulty rating and prerequisite skills. You can work on several new tricks within the same training session, and you may wish to keep a list of all your dog's tricks to train each session. Reinforcement is a constant process and just because your dog has mastered a trick doesn't mean you should stop practicing!

CAN ANY DOG LEARN TRICKS?

Sure! You'll find that the more tricks your dog knows, the quicker he'll pick up new ones. In a sense, you've taught him how to learn.

CUE, ACTION, REWARD

Teaching a trick comprises three parts, the first being a verbal or physical cue to your dog, signaling the desired behavior. The second part is the action performed by your dog, and the third is the reward. Do not attempt to bribe your dog by offering the reward before he has done the action, and do not expect your dog to perform an action before you have given the cue.

YOUR JOB AS A TRAINER

Your job as a trainer is to guide your dog in a consistent and motivating environment.

Guidance

Guide your dog through the process of executing a new behavior, rewarding baby steps along the way. The goal of each training session is to get better results than the last time.

Consistency

Know the behavior you are looking for, and don't be wishy-washy. Use the same voice and intonation each time you give a verbal cue and enunciate clearly.

Motivation

Think about an athletic coach. Is his job merely to plan the training schedule and tape it to the locker room door? No! He inspires, motivates, and encourages! He is upbeat when you are discouraged and slaps your shoulder with a "good job!" when you need it. You serve the same purpose for your dog. Every bit of enthusiasm you inject into your dog training will speed up his learning. And when your dog does something right use your high-pitched "happy voice" (yes, men, you have one too) to exude your delight!

TIMING

Imagine you are searching for something and are being guided by feedback of "hot" or "cold." But now imagine this feedback is being delayed before you hear it. You may actually be receiving "cold" feedback as you approach the object or vise versa. Not only is the object not being found, but you are getting frustrated at the inconsistency of the feedback. Imagine how much easier this task would be if the feedback were given with correct timing.

In trick training, it is imperative that you mark (with a word, treat, or clicker) the exact moment that your dog performed correctly. Don't reward 10 seconds later, as you may be rewarding a completely different behavior.

A common timing mistake is in rewarding too late. For example, you tell your dog to sit, and he does. You fish for a treat in your pocket, and he stands up to receive it. What did you just reward? You rewarded him for standing up! The treat should have been given while the dog was in the proper position—sitting. Always reward your dog while he is in the desired position.

MOTIVATORS/REWARDS

"Shouldn't my dog want to learn tricks merely to please me?" Dogs do, in general, want to please their owners—but learning is hard! Would you expect your child to do his homework every night merely to please you? Maybe, but a reward sure makes work more enticing ... whether it be a half hour of TV, or a nice liver treat!

A motivator, or reward, can come in different forms—a food morsel, favorite toy, clicker signal, or praise. In this book, the steps rely mostly on food treats. Food is enjoyed by all dogs, is quick to dispense and be swallowed, and is a clear way to signal a correct response. Keep your dog extra motivated when learning a new trick by using "people food" treats such as hot dogs, cheese, pizza crusts, noodles, meatballs, or whatever gets his mouth watering! During the beginning stages of learning, a toy can be a distraction, as it takes a while for you to take it back and get your dog to regain focus. Praise is great, but can be arbitrary and unclear ... "Good! No, wait, you moved, sort of... ." Use a small but tasty food treat to reward the desired behavior.

New dog trainers are always stingy with rewards. They attempt to reward with praise or regular dog kibble. Trick training, however, is dependent upon the dog's motivation and you want to make this activity the most fun thing he does all day! Go ahead, give 'em the good stuff!

For those experienced in the technique of clicker training, a clicker signal may be used to mark the correct behavior, followed by the treat.

Do I have to carry around treats for the rest of my life?

Before worrying about emptying our pockets of treats, we need to make the behavior an automatic response. No matter how it is achieved, if you tell your dog to "sit" 500 times, and he sits, it becomes an automatic response. For the first 500 times, he was sitting because you were tempting him with a treat. Later, however, his muscle memory just hears the word "sit" and does it! It is at this point that you can start weaning your dog off his expectation of a reward. Rather than weaning completely off treats, however, use them as sporadic rewards.

Upping the Ante

The purpose of a treat is to reward a good effort. In kindergarten, a child gets a gold star for printing her name. In first grade, she only gets a gold star if she prints it neatly, and in second grade cursive is required for that same reward. What may have earned your dog a treat in the past, may no longer be enough to earn that treat today. We call this "upping the ante." When first learning to shake a paw, reward your dog for barely lifting his paw, or for batting your hand. Once he has the hang of this, withhold the treat until he lifts his paw higher, or holds it longer. Every time your dog is achieving a step with about 75 percent success, up the ante and demand a higher skill to earn the treat.

Jackpot

We all know the lure of a jackpot. Having achieved it once, we will sit at the slot machine all night in hopes of being rewarded with that elusive prize. The jackpot theory, when applied to dog training, can be a more effective motivator than consistent rewards. Here's how to use it: ask your dog to perform some behaviors he is working on. If he does them fairly well, give him no reward or a small reward. When he performs a behavior very well or better than he has in the past, jackpot! Give him a whole handful of treats! Wow, will that make an impression on him! He will continue trying extra hard in hopes of hitting that jackpot again.

Along the same lines, using several different types of treats during a training session can keep your dog motivated— "maybe I'll get the hot dog this time!"

HELP YOUR DOG BE SUCCESSFUL

The key to keeping your dog motivated is to keep him challenged, achieving regular successes. Try not to let your dog be wrong more than two or three times in a row, or he could become discouraged and not wish to perform. Instead, go back to an easier step for a while.

PUT IN THE TIME

When teaching a new trick, it often appears that your dog is not getting the concept and has no idea what the desired behavior is. He'll be squirming and pawing and obsessing over the treat in your hand. You might feel as if he will never understand. Don't stress it. Go through the same motions day after day, and one day you'll see a lightbulb go off in his head. That's the moment that truly bonds you with your dog.

WHY PEOPLE FAIL

Picture this failure scenario: you tell your dog to spin, while luring him in a circle with your treat, just as this book instructs. Your dog squirms and nips at your hand. You raise your voice and say in a more firm tone, "spin!" Your dog scratches himself, ignoring you. You grab his collar, yelling this time "spin!" while you drag him in a circle. He cowers down, while you grumble about your dumb dog.

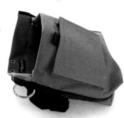

The single most common reason people fail teaching dog tricks is their lack of patience. Even trainers with bad timing, poor coordination, and lack of common sense can manage to teach tricks better than an impatient trainer.

Picture this success scenario: you tell your dog to spin, while luring him in a circle with your treat, just as this book instructs. Your dog squirms and nips at your hand. You try again, luring your dog in a circle, as before. Your dog scratches himself, ignoring you. You try again, and your dog performs a lopsided sort of spin. "Yeah! That was great!" You try again, and again, and again, and a few hundred more times ... and one day ... you have it! How lucky are you to have the world's smartest dog?

Progress can be slow and frustrating—keeping an even temper and consistent training method requires patience.

END ON A HIGH NOTE!

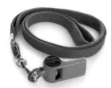

Practicing new tricks is mentally tiring for your dog. Keep it fun and end the session while your dog is still wanting more. End on a successful note, even if you have to go back to an easier behavior to achieve this.

LURING VERSUS MANIPULATING

There are two obvious ways to get a dog into a desired position: you can lure him by guiding him with a treat or toy, or you can assert physical pressure to manipulate him into position. It is tempting to manipulate your dog's body physically because it is faster and more precise, however it can actually delay the learning process. By manipulating your dog, you are encouraging him to relinquish initiative and be led. He is not required to engage his brain and is not learning the motor skills required to position his body by himself. When possible, it is always preferable to lure your dog to position his body himself.

USE "WHOOPS" INSTEAD OF "NO"

Trick training is the yin to obedience training's yang. Trick training allows the dog to be silly and encourages independent action. You want to keep the enthusiasm high during training sessions or your dog could shut down for fear of being wrong. Save the word "no" for when your dog is being naughty. If your dog is giving you an incorrect behavior, it is probably not intentional. Instead of "no," try a more lighthearted "whoops!"

FIRST PRAISE, THEN TOUCH, AND TREAT LAST

As discussed earlier, correct timing of your reward is essential. When teaching new tricks, food is often used as a lure and is released instantly to mark a correct behavior. For more general obedience training, or when rewarding your dog at the end of a session, reward in this order: praise, pat on the head, and then a food reward. Not only will this serve to keep your dog in a calm state of mind, but an association will develop whereby verbal praise will be pleasantly associated with your touch, and your touch will be associated with the food reward.

RELEASE WORD, "OK!"

Your dog needs to understand at which times he is under your control and at which times he has been released. When instructed to "down" or "stay" for example, your dog is expected to remain in that position until you release him with your release word. "OK" is the most commonly used release word. When a training session has ended, "OK" releases your dog to run and play. "OK" also releases your dog to jump out of the parked car, to pounce on a toy, and to play with another dog.

WHAT IS THE PURPOSE OF HAND SIGNALS?

Dogs can perform a trick based upon a verbal cue or hand signal. Hand signals are extremely useful for dogs performing in movies on quiet sets, and they generally give you more options. When a child asks your dog a question, your subtle "bark" hand signal can cue your dog to answer! Most dogs actually respond to hand signals more readily than verbal cues. Try it with your dog: use a verbal cue from one trick while signaling for another trick. Most often, the dog will perform the trick indicated by your hands!

CAN I MAKE UP MY OWN WORDS AND SIGNALS FOR TRICKS?

Words and signals for some tricks are more standardized than others. Basic obedience commands and many agility commands are widely used and have evolved with good reason. It can be helpful to use standardized verbal cues and hand signals, especially if your dog has aspirations of a movie career. Hand signals may look arbitrary but have often evolved from the methods used in a dog's initial training. The raising of the hand as a signal to "sit" evolves from your initial upward baiting when teaching the command. A downward hand motion is used to signal "down" and parallels your initial baiting of your dog near the floor. The toe-touch foot signal for "take a bow" draws your dog's attention toward the floor, coaxing his head downward. And the flick of your wrist to the right is a diminished version of the large circle you drew when teaching your dog to "spin."

Trick training, of course, is not a life-or-death pursuit and if you want to make up your own words and signals, nobody can stop you! A word of caution though: the more tricks you teach, the quicker you will run out of words. "Left" and "right" are tempting to use in the beginning, but a time may come when wish you had saved those words for a different trick.

CAN I MAKE UP MY OWN TRICKS?

Some of the best tricks happen by accident! If your dog acts out a long and laborious death in the "play dead" trick, capitalize on his inventiveness and teach the trick his way. In obedience class, your job is to instruct your dog on the correct behaviors, and his job is to do exactly what you wish. In trick training you are a team—allow the training process to be a collaborative one.

CHAINING COMMANDS

This is the really fun part! Once your dog has learned individual behaviors, you can chain them together and give a name to this new set of actions. "Night-night," for example, chains the behaviors of **come, down, take it, roll over,** and **head down** to produce an impressive trick of your dog rolling himself up in a blanket! There are many ways to use command chains, and even in practice they are a great brain exercise for your dog. Even a simple command of "target, sit" engages your dog's brain to execute first one action and then another.

HOW LONG DOES IT TAKE TO TRAIN A DOG?

How many years does it take for a child to become educated? For an athlete to become skilled? How many piano lessons until you're a musician? Dog training should

be thought of as a lifelong process. Although at some point your dog will be able to produce a behavior on cue, he will still need repetition and refinement to maintain and improve his skills. Challenge your dog with new skills for the rest of his life, and you'll find your bond will increase tenfold.

REALISTIC EXPECTATIONS

As you read the table of contents in this book, you may be having wonderful fantasies of lounging on the couch while your dog obediently gets you a beer from the fridge. Or perhaps you envision commanding your dog to help with the housework by gathering up all his toys into his toy box. Let me burst your bubble right now, your dog is never going do such complicated tricks completely independent of you, and certainly not without a reward. Tricks like these will require you to be within eye contact of your dog and will probably require verbal coaching and multiple commands. Remember, while these tricks mimic everyday simple human chores, they are complicated challenges for your dog.

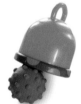

LET'S START TRAINING!

You're on your way to becoming the next great trick dog team. Grab your treat bag, Rover's favorite toy, your copy of *101 Dog Tricks*, and let's get started!

TOP 10 TRICK TRAINING TIPS:

1. Reward with tasty treats
2. Reward while your dog is in the correct position
3. Reward immediately (no fishing in pockets)
4. Train before dinner
5. Training comes before playtime
6. End the session with your dog wanting more
7. Be consistent
8. Motivate—use your happy voice
9. Be patient—it won't happen overnight
10. Be a fun person to be around

Chapter 1

Groundwork

"Obedience" is a word often misinterpreted in dog training to suggest the imposition of a dominating control over our dog. But let's get past the word and think of basic obedience skills as the groundwork upon which a successful living arrangement between dog and owner is achieved. The **sit**, **down**, **come**, and **stay** behaviors are marks of a civilized and well-behaved dog. These behaviors will also be required for almost every trick in this book, and time spent teaching them now will reduce frustration down the road.

"Since my dog already knows his groundwork commands, why should we continue to practice them?"

Consider this: the concert pianist warms up by playing scales, the olympic gymnast rolls summersaults, the teacher reviews lesson plans, and the NBA athlete works on his free throws.

Obedience training serves a greater purpose than merely teaching your dog to perform behaviors upon command. It is a mental exercise and a comfortable routine that allows you to reconnect with your dog. Warming up with these familiar skills gives your dog the confidence to achieve new ones.

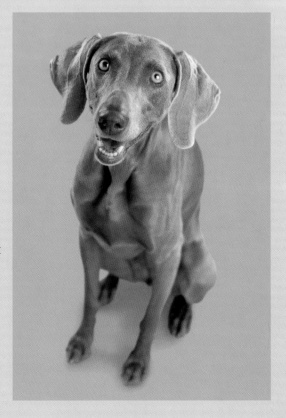

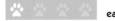

Sit

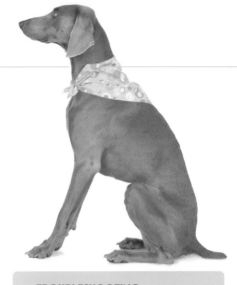

TEACH IT:

Your dog sits squarely on his hindquarters and remains there until released.

1 Stand or kneel in front of your dog, holding a treat in your hand a little higher than your dog's head.

2 Slowly move the treat straight back over your dog's head. This should cause his nose to point up and his rear to drop. If his rear does not drop, keep moving the treat straight backward toward his tail. The instant his rear touches the floor, release the treat and mark the behavior by saying "good sit!"

3 If your dog is not responding to the food lure, use your index finger and thumb to put pressure on either side of his haunches, just forward of his hip bones. Pull up on his leash at the same time to rock him back into a sit. Praise and reward him while he is sitting.

4 Once your dog is consistently sitting, wait a few seconds before rewarding. Remember to only reward while your dog is in the correct position—sitting.

WHAT TO EXPECT: Puppies as young as six weeks can start learning this command, and it is often the first trick a dog learns. Within a week, you should see some progress!

VERBAL CUE
Sit
HAND SIGNAL

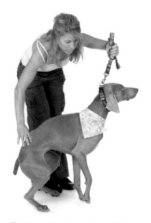

TROUBLESHOOTING

MY DOG JUMPS AT MY HAND WITH THE TREAT
Hold the treat lower, so that he can reach it while standing.

MY DOG SITS, BUT KEEPS GETTING UP
In a gentle but firm manner, keep placing your dog back in a **sit**. Once he has learned the behavior, he should not break his **sit** until released.

TIP! Command your dog to sit before each meal. This reinforces your position as pack leader and is just good manners!

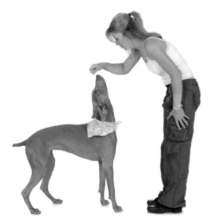

1 Hold a treat over your dog's head.

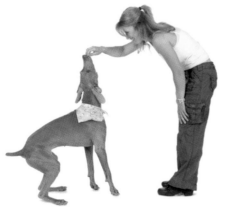

2 Move it straight back.

3 Press his haunches while pulling up on the leash.

Down

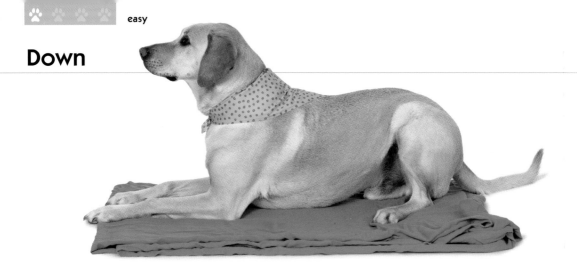

TROUBLESHOOTING

MY DOG IS RESISTANT TO THIS BEHAVIOR

Your dog lying down before you is interpreted as subservience to you. Evaluate your status as pack leader.

MY DOG DOESN'T STAY DOWN

If he stands up, don't reward him, and put him back down. Standing on his leash will cause him to self-correct if he tries to stand up.

MY DOG DOWNS IN ONE ROOM, BUT NOT ANOTHER

Pay attention to the ground surface. Short-coated dogs will often resist downing on hard floor. Try a carpet or towel.

BUILD ON IT! Once you've mastered **down**, it will be an easy step to learn **crawl** (page 144)!

TIP! When a dog jumps on you or the sofa, use the command "off" instead of "down."

TEACH IT:

Your dog drops to rest on either his chest and belly or askew on his hip. This vital command could help avert dangerous situations such as unsafe road crossings.

1. With your dog sitting facing you, hold a treat to his nose and lower it slowly to the floor.

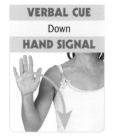

VERBAL CUE

Down

HAND SIGNAL

2. If you're lucky, your dog will follow the treat with his nose and lie down, at which time you can release the treat and praise him. Remember to only release the treat while your dog is in the correct position—lying down. If your dog slouches instead of lying down, slide the treat slowly toward him on the floor between his front paws or away from him. It may take a little time but your dog should eventually lie down.

3. If your dog is not responding to the food lure, put slight pressure on his shoulder blade, pushing down and to the side. Praise your dog when he drops to the floor. It is always preferable to coax the dog to position himself without your physical manipulation.

4. Once your dog is consistently lying down, gradually delay the release of the treat. With your dog lying down, say "wait, wait" and then "good" and release the treat. Varying the time before treating will keep your dog focused. The dog should not move from the down position until you have given your release word, "OK!"

WHAT TO EXPECT: Herding breeds and sedentary or massive dogs often drop easier into a **down** position than long-legged, deep-chested, and hyper dogs. This skill can be learned by dogs and puppies of any age.

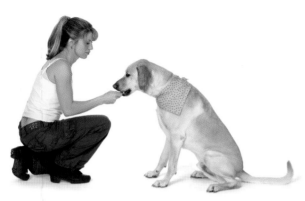

1 Hold a treat to your dog's nose.

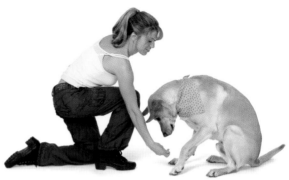

2 Lower the treat to the floor.

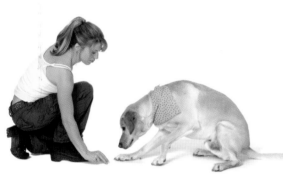

Slide the treat toward or away from him.

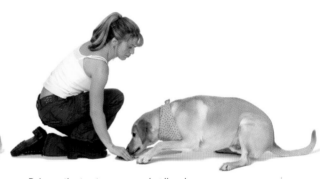

Release the treat once your dog lies down.

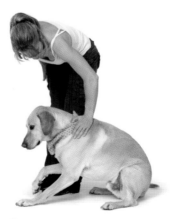

3 Press downward and to the side.

Stay

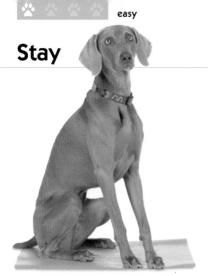

TEACH IT:

When in a **stay**, your dog holds his current position until released.

1 Start with your dog sitting or lying down, as he is less likely to move from these positions. Use a leash to guarantee control. Stand directly in front of him and in a serious tone, say "stay," holding your palm flat, almost touching his nose.

VERBAL CUE
Stay
HAND SIGNAL

2 Move a short distance away, keeping eye contact with your dog, and return to him. Praise him with "good stay" and give him a treat. Be sure to give the praise and treat while your dog remains in the seated and staying position.

3 If your dog moves from his **stay** before you have released him, gently but firmly put him back in the spot where he was originally told to stay.

4 Gradually increase the time you ask your dog to stay, as well as the distance between yourselves. You want your dog to be successful so if he is breaking his stays, go back to a time and distance he is able to achieve.

WHAT TO EXPECT: The tone of your voice and your body language will be a big part of getting your message across. Be firm and consistent, and it won't take may sessions before your dog begins to understand.

TROUBLESHOOTING

MY DOG KEEPS GETTING UP

Use very little verbal communication when teaching this skill. Talking evokes action, and you want inaction. Solid body language will convey your seriousness.

MY DOG SEEMS TO BREAK HIS STAY A SECOND BEFORE I RELEASE HIM

Do not show him the treat until you give it to him, as it may pull him forward. Vary your pattern; sometimes return to him and leave him again without rewarding.

TIP! "Stay" means: don't move a muscle until I release you. "Wait" is less formal, meaning: stay approximately there for a short time. "Wait until I gather my things before jumping out of the car."

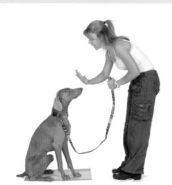

1 Command your dog to "stay."

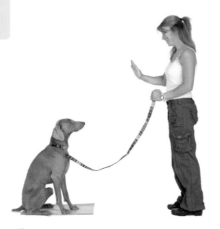

2 Move a short distance away.

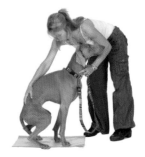

3 Return him to the original spot if he breaks.

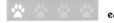 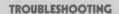 *easy*

Come

TEACH IT:

Upon your command, your dog **comes** immediately to you. In competition, this command ends with your dog sitting in front of you. In order for this command to be consistently obeyed, your status as pack leader needs to be definite. Always reward your dog for obeying your "come" command, whether it be with praise or a treat. Not obeying this command, however, should be viewed as a major infraction and should end with you physically bringing your dog to the spot from where you originally called him.

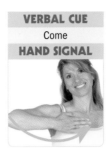

VERBAL CUE
Come
HAND SIGNAL

1 With your dog on a 6' (1.8 m) lead, command him to "come" and reel him quickly in to you, where he will be praised. Your command should sound happy, but firm. Give the command only once.

2 As your dog improves, graduate to a longer lead.

3 When you are ready to practice off-lead, do it in a fenced area. Let your dog drag a leash. If he does not obey your first command, go to him and firmly lead him back to the spot where you gave the command. Do not give a reward if the dog does not perform the command on his own, the first time you call. Put the long lead back on him and require him to do five successful "comes" before attempting off-lead again.

WHAT TO EXPECT: A dog can learn the meaning of the word very quickly, but the practice and enforcement of this command should continue for life.

TROUBLESHOOTING

ONCE OFF LEAD MY DOG RUNS OFF!
Do not chase your dog, as that will only encourage him. Stand your ground and demand that he come. Dogs respond to a leader.

DO I HAVE TO ENFORCE THIS COMMAND EVERY TIME I USE IT?
Yes. If you are not in a position to enforce it, don't give the command. Instead just call your dog's name or use "c'mon boy!"

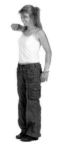

TIP! Call your dog to **come** for good things. Never call "come" for a bath or trip to the vet—go and get your dog instead.

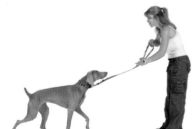

1 Reel your dog in to you.

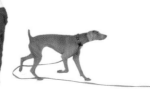

2 Move to a longer lead.

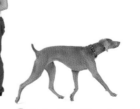

3 Train off-lead in a fenced area.

Chapter 2
Traditional Favorites

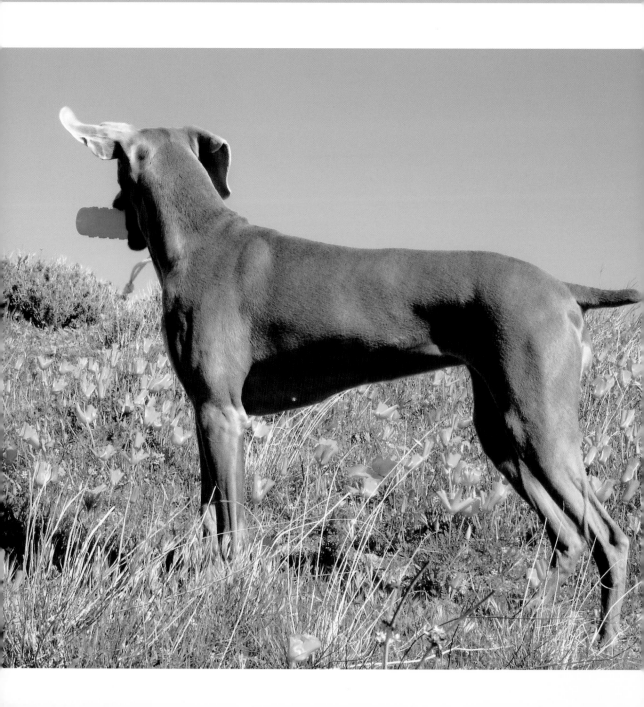

Fetch, shake, speak, and play dead … these useful, useless, and always charming tricks have been around since cavemen first shared their bones with wolves. Regardless of a lack of titles after his name, a dog who falls to the ground on the command of "bang" or offers a polite paw to his guests will be top dog among your friends! These tricks are expected of dogs and it is your task, possibly even your duty, to teach them to your clever canine.

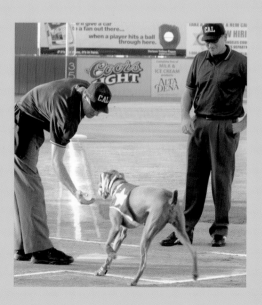

The tricks in this chapter have withstood the test of time for a reason: they are simple to teach and easy to learn. They capitalize on dogs' natural behaviors by associating familiar actions with verbal cues. Is your dog vocal? It should be simple for you to elicit a bark, associate it with a cue, and reward it. Retrievers will no doubt fetch before they are out of puppyhood, and hyper dogs will be excited to proffer a paw when encouraged to "shake." Let's get started teaching these traditional favorites!

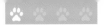
Shake Hands—Left and Right

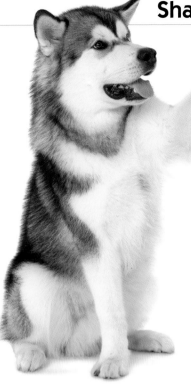

TEACH IT:

When **shaking hands**, your polite pooch raises his paw to chest height, allowing guests to shake his paw. This skill is taught for both paws.

VERBAL CUE

Shake (left paw)
Paw (right paw)

HAND SIGNAL

1. With your dog sitting before you, hide a treat in your right hand, low to the ground. Encourage your dog to paw at it by saying "get it" and "shake." Reward your dog with the treat the moment his left paw comes off the ground.

2. Gradually raise the height of your hand, upping the ante, until he is lifting his paw to chest height.

3. Transition to using the hand signal. Stand up and hold the treat in your left hand, behind your back, and extend your right hand while cuing "shake." When your dog paws your extended hand, support his paw in the air while you reward him with the treat from behind your back.

4. Repeat these steps on the opposite side to teach "paw."

WHAT TO EXPECT: Any dog can learn this trick, and it's always an endearing gesture. Practice a couple of times per day, and always leave off on a high note. Chain these behaviors together to alternate "shake" and "paw" in quick succession.

TROUBLESHOOTING

INSTEAD OF PAWING AT MY HAND, MY DOG NOSES IT

Bop his nose a little to discourage this. He may try barking, nuzzling, or doing nothing. Be patient, and keep encouraging him. If he is not lifting his paw on his own, tap or barely lift it for him and then reward.

BUILD ON IT! Once you've mastered **shake hands** and **paw**, use a similar action to learn **chorus line kicks** (page 176) and **wave goodbye** (page 202).

TIP! Use the word "good" to mark the exact instant your dog performed the desired behavior.

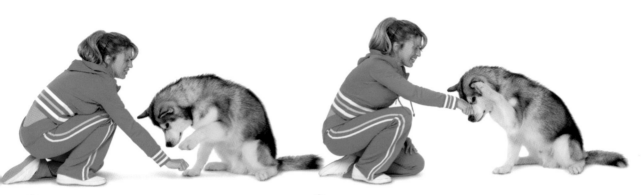

1 Hide a treat in your right hand, low to the ground.

2 As your dog improves, raise your hand.

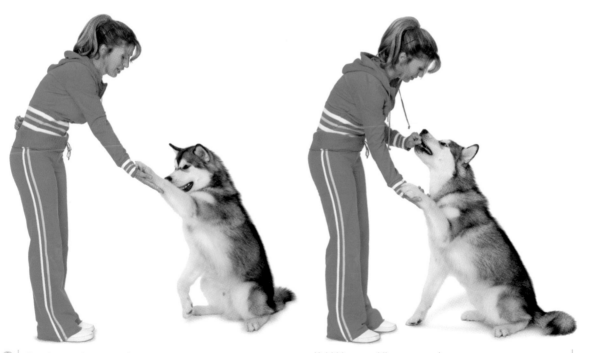

3 Stand up and cue your dog.

Hold his paw while you reward.

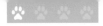

Fetch/Take It

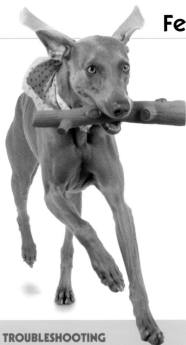

TEACH IT:

In **fetch**, your dog is directed to retrieve a specified object. **Take it** is when he takes an object within reach into his mouth.

FETCH:

1. Use a box cutter to make a 1" (2.5 cm) slit in a tennis ball. Show your dog as you drop a treat inside the ball.

2. Toss the ball playfully and encourage the dog to bring it back to you by patting your legs, acting excited, or running from him.

3. Take the ball from your dog and squeeze it to release the treat for him. As he is unable to get the treat himself, he will learn to bring it to you for his reward.

VERBAL CUE
Fetch (retrieval)
Take it
(object within reach)

TAKE IT:

1. Select a toy that your dog enjoys and playfully hand it to him while giving the verbal cue.

2. Have him hold it only a few seconds before removing it from his mouth and trading him a treat for it. As your dog improves, extend the time he holds the object before treating. Only treat if you remove the toy from your dog's mouth, not if he drops it on his own.

3. Be creative! Have your dog hold a flag as he circles the field or have him carry a charming "feed me" sign. A dog holding a pipe is always good for a laugh, and a posh pooch carrying a basket of cocktail napkins is sure to impress!

WHAT TO EXPECT: Many dogs are natural retrievers and will understand this trick within a few days.

TROUBLESHOOTING

MY DOG HAS NO INTEREST IN CHASING THE BALL

Motivate your dog by acting excited and chasing the ball yourself. Bat it around or bounce it off walls. Make it a competition and race him for it.

MY DOG GETS THE BALL AND RUNS OFF WITH IT

Never chase your dog when he is playing keep-away. Lure him back with a treat, or run away from him to encourage him to chase you. Have a second ball to get his attention.

BUILD ON IT! Once you've mastered **fetch**, build on it with: **fetch my slippers** (page 36), **newspaper delivery** (page 40), and **directed retrieve** (page 184). Build on **take it** with: **carry my purse** (page 44).

TIP! Excessive mouthing of tennis balls can lead to tooth wear. If your dog is a chewer, give him a hard rubber toy such as a Kong.

FETCH:

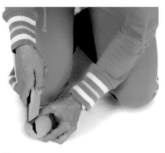 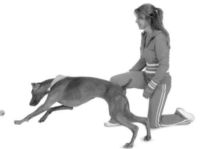 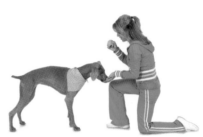

1 Make a slit in a tennis ball and drop a treat inside.

2 Toss the ball playfully.

3 Squeeze the ball to release the treat.

TAKE IT:

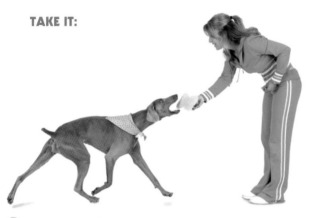 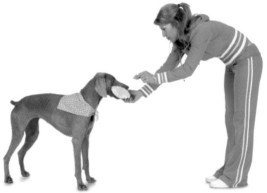

1 Hand your dog a favorite toy.

2 Trade him a treat for the toy.

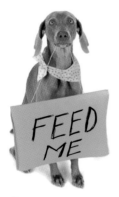

3 Have your dog take and hold other objects!

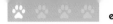

Drop It/Give

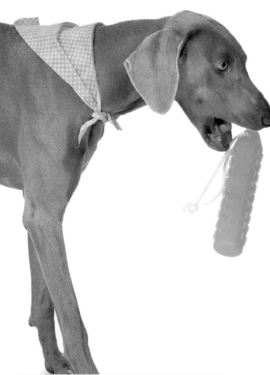

TEACH IT:

On the **drop it** cue, your dog releases the object from his mouth, dropping it onto the ground. **Give** is released to your hand.

DROP IT:

1 Is your dog food or toy motivated? Point to the ground and command your dog to "drop it." Do not move from your location, and keep repeating the command. It may take several minutes, but when your dog finally drops the toy, reward him with food or by throwing his toy.

GIVE:

1 While your dog has a toy in his mouth, tell him to "give" and offer him a treat in exchange for the toy. He will have to release the toy to eat the treat, at which time you can praise him.

2 Give your dog his toy back, so he understands that relinquishing it to you does not mean that it will be taken away.

WHAT TO EXPECT: Dogs vary on their willingness to relinquish a toy. Build a habit of only throwing the toy if your dog relinquishes it willingly.

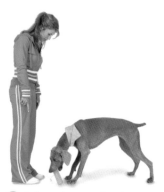

DROP IT: 1 Point to the ground and command "drop it."

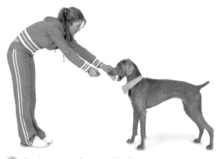

GIVE: 1 Trade a treat for your dog's toy.

TROUBLESHOOTING

MY DOG WILL NOT RELEASE THE TOY
Try using a less desirable toy and rewarding him with a highly desired toy when he obeys.

SHOULD I FORCE AN OBJECT AWAY FROM HIM?
No, as this could result in a dog bite, intentional or not. A better way to get a dog to release his grip is to pull upward on the skin on the side of his rib cage.

BUILD ON IT! Once you've mastered **drop it**, build on it with **tidy up your toys** (page 46), and **basketball** (page 90).

TIP! To open a dog's mouth for exam, put your hand over the top of his muzzle, roll his lips over his teeth, and separate the jaws.

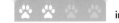
Balance and Catch

TEACH IT:

Your dog balances a treat or toy placed on his nose and, at your signal, tosses it and makes the catch.

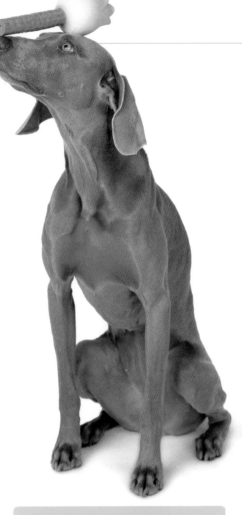

1 Position your dog in a **sit** (page 15) facing you. Gently hold your dog's muzzle parallel to the floor and place a treat upon the bridge of his nose. In a low voice, coach him to "waaaait."

VERBAL CUE
Wait, Catch

2 Hold this position for just a few seconds before releasing his muzzle and telling him to "catch!" Exuberant dogs will probably send the treat flying, and will have to chase it down. You'll want to slow these dogs down by using a calm, quiet "catch." Practice will hone their abilities until they can do it every time.

3 If your dog is allowing the treat to fall to the floor, pretend to race him to pick it up. He will learn that he needs to catch the treat or risk losing it to you on the floor.

4 As your dog improves, require him to balance the treat on his nose without the help of your hand on his muzzle. Placing the treat near the end of your dog's nose is usually easiest to catch, but every dog is different.

WHAT TO EXPECT: Some dogs will have naturally better coordination, but all dogs will benefit from the motor functions practiced in this skill.

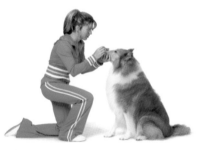

1 Hold his muzzle parallel and place a treat upon it.

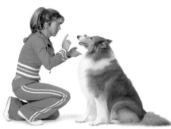

4 Remove your hand while he balances the treat.

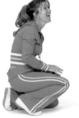

Practice will perfect his catch!

TROUBLESHOOTING

HIS NOSE IS TOO SHORT!
Although it is possible to teach this trick to pug-nosed breeds, it is more difficult. A bendable treat, such as a wet noodle, is easier to balance.

THE TREAT FLIES THROUGH THE AIR WHEN MY DOG TRIES TO CATCH IT
Here's another case where you can race him for the treat to increase his motivation to catch it quickly.

BUILD ON IT! Increase the difficulty of this trick by having your dog **beg** (page 28) while balancing the treat.

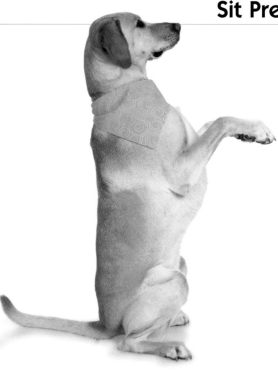

Sit Pretty/Beg

TEACH IT:

When "please" doesn't work ... it may be time to beg! From a sitting position, your dog raises his forequarters while keeping his rear on the floor. Your dog should sit on both hindquarters, with a straight spine, paws tucked into his chest. The alignment of his hindquarters, thorax, forequarters, and head is key to his balance.

SMALL DOGS:

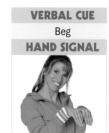

VERBAL CUE
Beg
HAND SIGNAL

1. Position your dog in a **sit** (page 15), facing you. Use a treat to lure his head up and back, while cueing him to "beg." Allow him to nibble the treat from your fist, to entice him to stay in this position. If his hindquarters lift off the floor, lower your treat a little, tell him to sit, and tap his bottom down.

2. As your dog's balance improves, move away and use the verbal cue and hand signal. After several seconds, toss the treat to your dog. Remember to reward your dog while he is in the correct position, not after he has lowered his front paws.

BIG DOGS:

1. Position your dog in a sit. Stand directly behind him, with your heels together and toes pointed apart.

2. Use a treat to guide his head back and straight up, until he is upright. Steady his chest with your other hand. He will need to find his balance; as he improves, use a lighter touch on his back and chest.

WHAT TO EXPECT: Some dogs may learn this behavior easily, while others have a much harder time establishing their balance. This trick builds thigh and lower back strength, which will benefit any dog. Your dog will sit up and beg for your praise!

"My favorite things to roll in: wet grass, horse manure, kitty's hairballs."

TROUBLESHOOTING

MY DOG JUMPS AT THE TREAT
Move slower when positioning your hand. Do not reward your dog if he jumps.

MY DOG STANDS UP ON HIS HIND LEGS
Keep your hand lower, and gently say "sit." Hold the treat at face level.

MY DOG CAN'T SEEM TO BALANCE
This trick is easier for small dogs and round dogs. Large, long, and deep-chested dogs can learn to beg, but they need more time to find their balance.

BUILD ON IT! Now that your dog is comfortable balancing, try teaching him to stand or walk on his hind legs!

TIP! Set small dogs on a table for easy access while training.

SMALL DOGS:

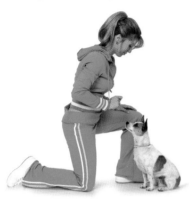 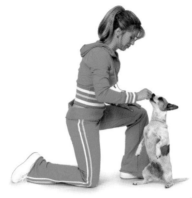 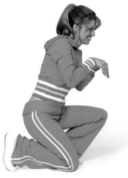

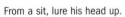

1 From a sit, lure his head up.   Allow him to nibble the treat.   **2** As balance improves, move away.

BIG DOGS:

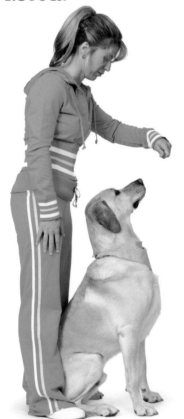 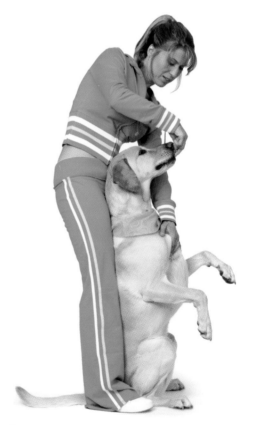

1 Position your heels behind your dog, with your toes pointed apart.

2 Steady his chest while you lure him up.

Speak

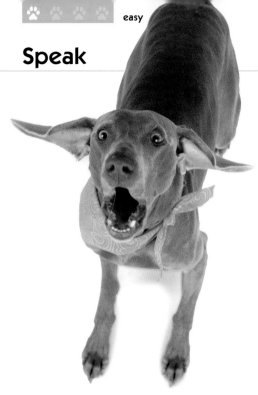

TEACH IT:

Your dog barks on cue. If your dog is barking up the wrong tree ... then this is the trick for him!

1. Observe what causes your dog to bark—a doorbell or knock, the postman, the sight of you with his leash—and use that stimulus to teach this trick. Because most dogs bark at the sound of a doorbell, we'll use that as an example. Stand at your front door, with the door open so your dog will be able to hear the bell. Give the cue "bark" and press the doorbell. When your dog barks, immediately reward him and reinforce the cue with "good bark." Repeat this about six times.

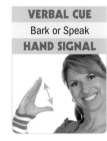

VERBAL CUE
Bark or Speak
HAND SIGNAL

2. Continuing in the same session, give the cue but don't ring the bell. You may have to cue several times to get a bark. If your dog is not barking, return to the previous step.

3. Try this trick in a different room. Strangely enough, this can be a difficult transition for your dog. If at any point your dog is repeatedly unsuccessful, return to the previous step.

WHAT TO EXPECT: Provided you've got a reliable stimulus that causes your dog to bark, he can learn this trick in one session.

TROUBLESHOOTING

I'VE CREATED A BARKING MONSTER!
Never reward your dog for a bark unless you asked for this behavior. Otherwise he'll speak up anytime he wants something!

I CAN'T FIND A STIMULUS TO MAKE MY DOG BARK.
Dogs will often bark out of frustration. Tease him with a treat: "Do you want it? Speak for it!"

BUILD ON IT! Once you've mastered **speak**, use this skill to learn **my dog can count** (page 180)!

TIP! Lower your voice, with your finger to your lips, and tell your dog to "speak, whisper." Reward a low volume sound.

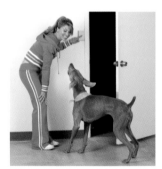

1. Ring the doorbell.

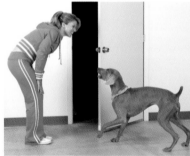

2. Try to elicit the behavior with only the verbal cue.

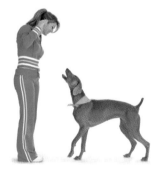

3. Change locations and cue your dog.

Roll Over

TEACH IT:

Your dog rolls sideways on his back, completing a full rotation.

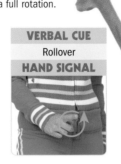

VERBAL CUE
Rollover
HAND SIGNAL

1 Start with your dog in a **down** (page 16) position, facing you. Kneel down in front of him, holding a treat to the side of his head opposite the direction you wish him to roll.

2 Move the treat from his nose toward his shoulder blade while telling him to "roll over." This should lure your dog to roll on his side. Praise and release the treat.

3 When you are ready to move to the next step, continue the motion with your hand as you move the treat from his shoulder blade toward his backbone. This should lure him to roll onto his back, and over to his other side. Reward the moment he lands on his opposite side.

4 As he improves, use a more subtle hand gesture.

WHAT TO EXPECT: Practice five to ten times per session, and in two weeks your dog could be rolling over on cue!

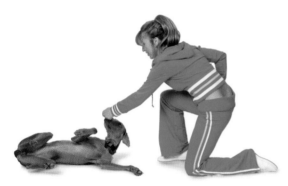

2 Lure his nose toward his shoulder blade.

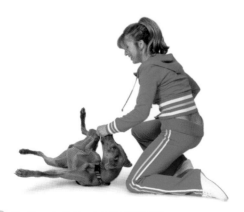

3 Continue luring toward his backbone.

TROUBLESHOOTING

MY DOG IS SQUIRMING, BUT NOT ROLLING ONTO HIS SIDE

It's all about your hand position. You want his neck arched as if his nose were trying to touch his shoulder blade. Try not to physically push him to his side, as he may interpret this as a domineering action and submit.

MY DOG ROLLS TO HIS SIDE, BUT DOES NOT CONTINUE TO ROLL ONTO HIS BACK

In this case, help your your dog finish the rollover by gently guiding his front legs over with your hand.

BUILD ON IT! Build on this skill to teach **roll yourself in a blanket** (page 48).

TIP! Most dogs have a dominant side, so start by teaching a rollover in the direction your dog seems to prefer.

Play Dead

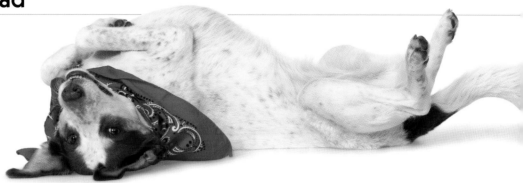

PREREQUISITES
Stay (page 18)
Roll over (page 31)

TROUBLESHOOTING

DEAD DOGS SHOULDN'T HAVE WAGGING TAILS!
Try lowering your voice to a more commanding tone to stop the wagging. Or don't worry about it ... it's sure to get a giggle!

MY DOG DOES A SLOW AGONIZING DEATH THAT REQUIRES SEVERAL BULLETS AND A FEW CIRCLES
Improvise with "darn, missed him! Will you die already! Talk about a scene stealer!"

TIP! As the use of a "finger gun" is not always appropriate with young children, consider using a command of "boo!" and scaring your dog to death instead.

"Things I don't like: baths, kitty sleeping in my bed, being left alone."

TEACH IT:

When **playing dead**, your dog rolls onto his back with his legs in the air. He remains "dead" until you cue his miraculous recovery. Stick 'em up or you're a dead dog!

1 Teach this trick after your dog has had some exercise and is ready to rest. Put your dog in a **down** (page 16) and kneel in front of him. Hold a treat to the side of his head and move it toward his shoulder blade, as you did when teaching **roll over** (page 31). Your dog should fall to his side.

VERBAL CUE
Bang
HAND SIGNAL

2 Continue to roll him to his back by guiding his midsection. Praise him and give him a belly scratch while he is on his back. Reinforce the verbal cue by saying "good bang."

3 As your dog improves, try to lure him into position with the treat only, without touching him. If he is likely to roll completely over instead of stopping half way, stop him with your hand on his chest, and then slowly release your grip so that he holds the position on his own.

4 Practice this skill until you are able to elicit the behavior with the "bang!" cue and hand signal. Your dog should stay in this position until he is released with "OK" or "you are healed!" or some other release word.

WHAT TO EXPECT: This position can be a little awkward for your dog, and will take some getting used to. Practice in combination with **roll over**, so your dog understands the difference.

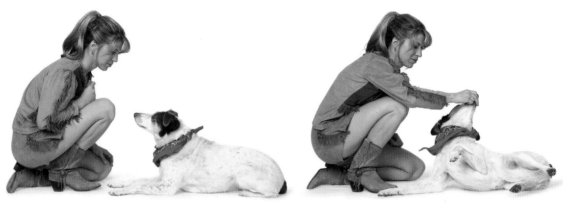

1 Put your dog in a down, facing you.

Lure him onto his side, as in a rollover.

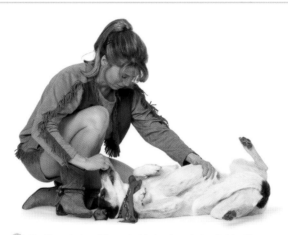

2 Continue to lure him onto his back and steady him there.

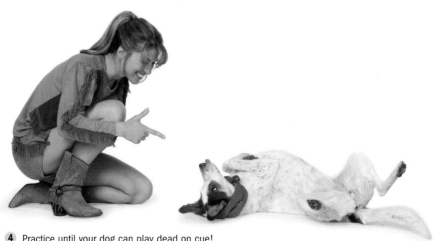

4 Practice until your dog can play dead on cue!

Chapter 3

Time for Chores

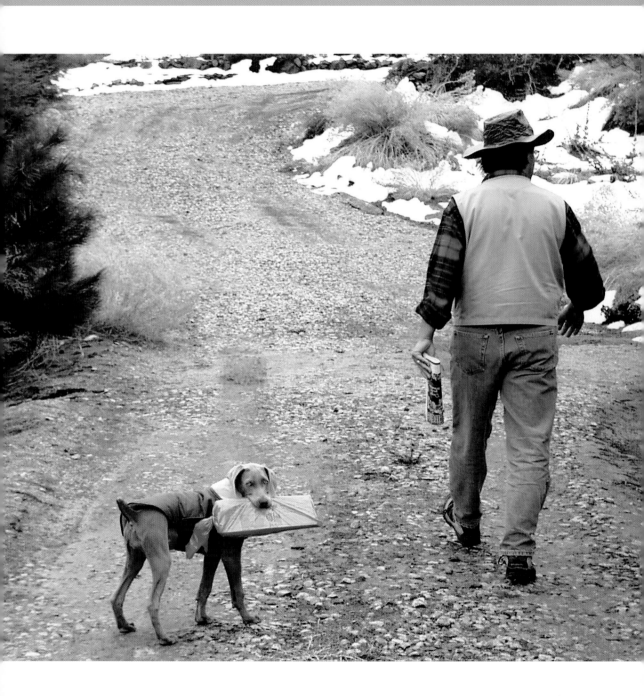

Dogs

and people have lived in symbiotic relationships throughout history, each providing the other with valuable services. People provide food, shelter, and veterinary care, while dogs traditionally served humans by offering protection, hunting assistance, flock tending, vermin control, and transportation by carts and sleds. In today's modern world, your dog may not be expected to serve in these traditional capacities, but that doesn't mean he gets a free ride! Your dog can still earn his keep by helping around the house with these modern chores.

Dogs need something to do. They want to feel useful and love to work for praise and a sense of accomplishment. In this chapter, you'll learn some useful tricks that can become part of your dog's daily chores. Sure, it will take effort to teach your dog, but think of the time you'll save each day when your dog fetches your morning newspaper, brings your slippers, and tidies up his toys into his toy box! (Feel free to try these out on your kids.)

Your dog will be most enthusiastic to do his chores if he feels they are important jobs. When he brings you the morning paper, take a moment to appreciate this wonderful service instead of casually tossing the paper on the table. When he carries your purse, don't let him get away with dropping or chewing it. This is a valuable item! And if he proudly offers you two slippers from different pairs go ahead and wear them with pride! After all, what's more important than the feelings of your best friend?

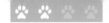
Fetch My Slippers

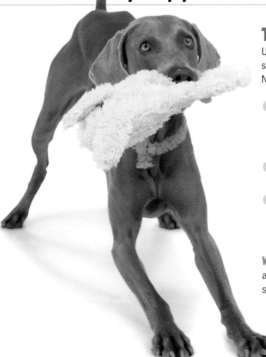

TEACH IT:

Upon your command, your dog will search for and bring one of your shoes. Your dog will distinguish between your shoes and someone else's. Note though, it is not guaranteed that you will receive a matching set!

1. In an empty environment, place one of your slippers a short distance from your dog. Point to the slipper, and tell your dog to "**fetch** shoe" (page 24). Reward a successful fetch.

VERBAL CUE

Fetch shoe

2. After several successful iterations, put the slipper out of site, or in another room, and send your dog to find it.

3. Once your dog is conditioned to retrieve one specific shoe, repeat the exercise with a different shoe. Your dog will come to understand that a "shoe" is any footwear that smells like you.

WHAT TO EXPECT: Practice this for as long as it is fun for your dog, about 4–6 times per session. In two weeks, you could be receiving slippers while sitting in your armchair!

PREREQUISITES
Fetch (page 24)

TROUBLESHOOTING

MY DOG BRINGS OTHER OBJECTS (TOYS, CLOTHES) INSTEAD OF MY SHOE
Your dog is excited and remembers he wants to bring you something... but can't remember what. Don't accept the object, but rather encourage him again to "fetch shoe."

MY DOG BROUGHT ME TWO SHOES... BUT FROM DIFFERENT SETS!
What can I say, either be happy with what you got or do a better job of cleaning up your clothes!

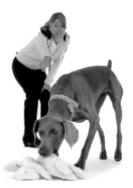

1. Instruct your dog to fetch.

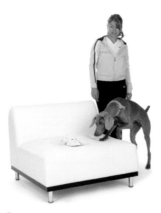

2. Put the slipper in another room.

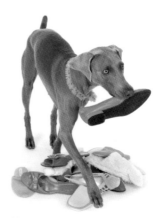

3. Repeat with a different shoe.

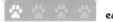
Get Your Leash

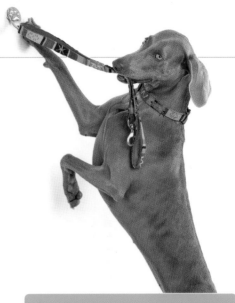

TEACH IT:

Your dog will fetch his leash from it's regular spot, either upon your command or whenever he wants to go for a walk.

1 Introduce the word "leash" to your dog by using it each time you put it on him. Toss his leash playfully and tell him to "**fetch** leash" (page 24). You'll want to secure the metal clasp within the leash so your dog doesn't bonk himself in the head with it in his exuberance! Forming a circle with the leash by buckling the clasp onto the handle is not always a good idea, as the dog can get tangled in the loop.

> **VERBAL CUE**
>
> Get your leash

2 Now put the leash in its regular spot, such as on a hook by the door. Point to it and encourage your dog to "get your leash!" Maneuvering the leash off the hook may be a little tricky, so be ready to help coax it off if your dog is having trouble. Reward your dog by immediately buckling his leash to his collar and taking him out for a walk. In this trick, the reward is a walk instead of a treat, so be sure to introduce this concept early on.

3 The next time you are ready to go for a walk, get your dog excited to go out, and then have him get his leash before leaving.

WHAT TO EXPECT: Don't be surprised if your dog interrupts your TV show by dropping his leash in your lap! This method of communicating his wishes sure beats barking and scratching at the door, so try to reward his politeness with a walk as often as possible.

> **PREREQUISITES**
> Fetch (page 24)

> **TROUBLESHOOTING**
>
> **SOMETIMES THE LEASH GETS STUCK ON THE WALL HOOK**
> An excited dog can pull the hook right out of the wall! A straight peg is a better idea.

> **BUILD ON IT!** Use the leash to teach **walk the dog**! (page 38)

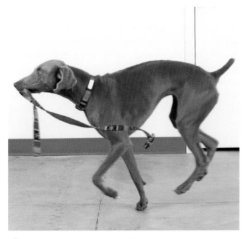

1 Introduce the word "leash" to your dog.

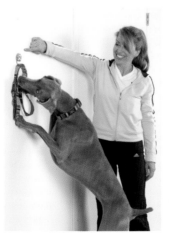

2 Have your dog take his leash from its normal spot.

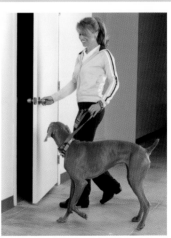

Reward your dog by taking him for a walk.

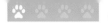
Walk the Dog

TROUBLESHOOTING

MY DOG DROPS THE LEASH WHEN HE IS BORED
Immediately pull your dog back to heel position and instruct him to "take it" again. He should not be allowed to drop the leash except upon your command.

THE DOGS SHOW AGGRESSION WHEN I ASK ONE TO HOLD THE LEASH OF THE OTHER
Don't put your dogs in this situation if you suspect there will be aggression. This wouldn't be the best way to work out pack-dominance issues.

BUILD ON IT! Learn **mail carrier** (page 76) to vary this trick by having one dog "deliver" the other dog to a family member!

TIP! The ideal leash length is 18"–24" (46–61 cm) longer than the distance from your waist to your dog's collar. A flat braided leather leash will become a favorite.

"I pull on my leash when I go for walks. Sometimes, people tell my owner she should train me."

TEACH IT:

This adorable trick is not so much useful as it is amusing. You'll be sure to get double takes as you stroll the block with your dutiful pooch as he walks himself. With your dog leashed, he carries the loop end of the leash in his mouth. Now that's doggoned clever!

① Fold up your dog's leash and secure it with a rubber band. Instruct your dog to "**take it**" (page 24). After a few moments, take the leash from his mouth and reward him.

② Practice **heeling** (page 160) with the folded leash in his mouth.

③ Now clip the leash to his collar and hand him just the loop end of the leash. Instruct him to take it and heel by your side. He's walking himself!

④ Clip the leash on another friendly dog and instruct both dogs to heel.

WHAT TO EXPECT: Your dog will have a new leash on life as he takes himself for walks. Dogs skilled in "take it" will pick this trick up quickly. The problem will be in convincing your dog to hold the leash for an extended time, especially when there are tempting smells to sniff. Your dog will enjoy the freedom of holding his own leash, and may even test your rules by trying to take the leash from your hand as you walk. This is dangerous territory, as it could be perceived as a challenge to your dominance. Give it some thought beforehand.

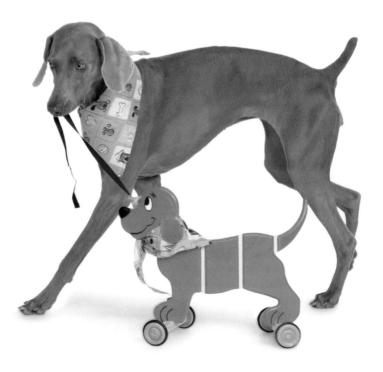

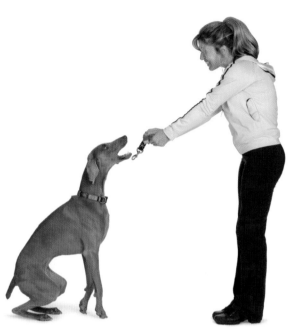

1 Fold his leash and have your dog "take it."

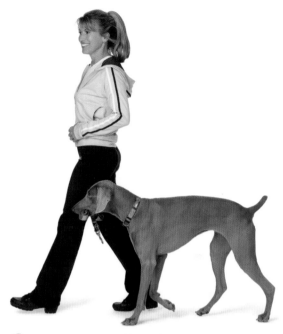

2 Heel with the leash in his mouth.

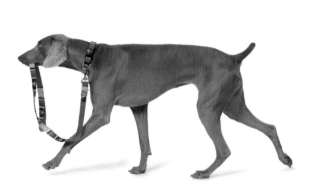

3 Attach the leash to his collar and have him take the loop end.

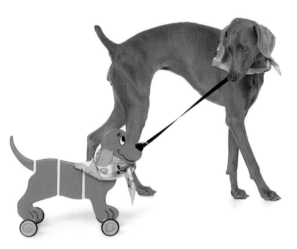

4 Teach one of your dogs to take the other for a walk!

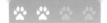

Newspaper Delivery

TROUBLESHOOTING

MY NEWSPAPER COMES FOLDED, NOT BAGGED, AND FALLS APART AS MY DOG CARRIES IT

Yep, that happens. Ask your delivery person to install a dog-height newspaper mailbox.

THERE'S DOG SLOBBER ON THE FRONT PAGE!

Large-jowled dogs such as bloodhounds and Newfoundlands are generous with their saliva! If your dog enjoys this job, walk out with him and wrap a section of yesterday's paper around the the new paper. Most of the salivation happens as dogs approach the front door, so be quick to take that paper!

TIP! Once your dog has learned to get the paper, don't pick it up for him if he drops it. It is now his responsibility.

TEACH IT:

Your dog will learn to bring the newspaper from the driveway or mailbox to your front door.

1 Roll up a section of the newspaper and secure it with a rubber band or masking tape. Toss it playfully indoors, and instruct your dog to "**fetch!** (page 24) Get the paper!" Do not allow him to shake or tear it, and reward each successful fetch.

VERBAL CUE
Get the paper

2 Now try it outside, tossing the paper in its usually delivery spot, while you stand nearby.

3 Gradually work your way back, so the paper is tossed in the same spot, but you are standing closer and closer to your front door. Give your dog the verbal cue and reward him with a treat or praise for retrieving the paper.

4 Now that your dog is competent in paper delivery, make it more challenging by hiding the paper in the bushes, as your paper boy does. If your mailbox has a flap door, your dog can learn to **pull it open** (page 73), **close it** (page 70), and even lower the flag (adapted from **turn off the light** page 68)!

WHAT TO EXPECT: Most dogs enjoy carrying things in their mouths, and will especially enjoy this daily task because of its importance! As dogs have a habit of dropping items after they lose interest, be consistent in teaching them that the paper is an object that needs to be reliably delivered.

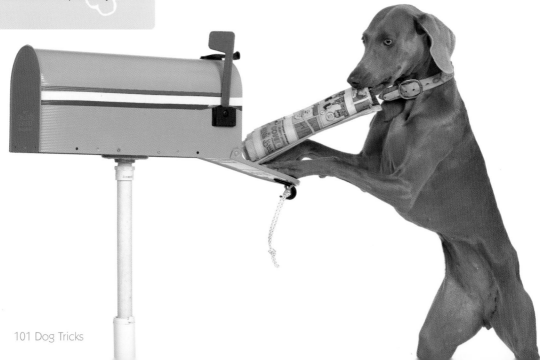

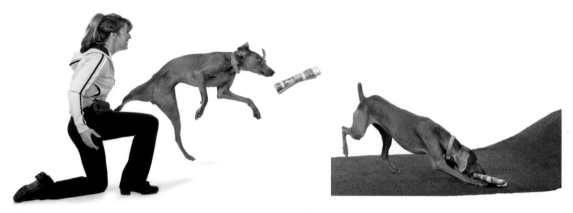

1 Secure the newspaper with a rubber band and practice fetching.

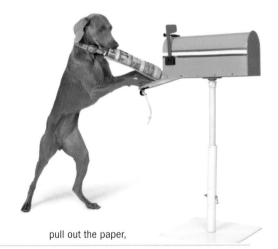

2 Toss the paper outdoors, in its usual delivery spot.

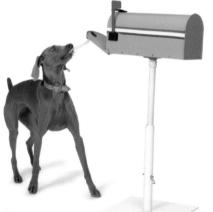

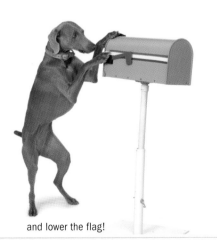

4 Teach your dog to open your mailbox,

pull out the paper,

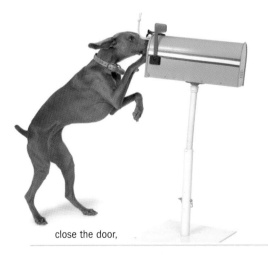

close the door,

and lower the flag!

Say Your Prayers

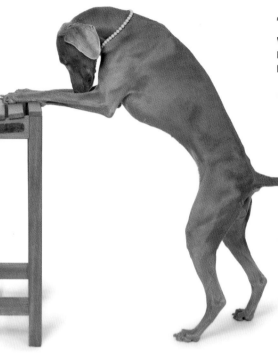

TEACH IT:

When **saying his prayers**, your dog places his front paws on the edge of a bed or chair, lowers his forequarters as in a bow, and hides his head between his arms.

1. Kneeling sideways in front of your dog, cue him to put his **paws on your arm** (page 198). When you reward this behavior, do so with a treat from your other hand positioned between your dog's paws, so that he must bow his head for the treat. Start by requiring only a mild bowing of his head, and be sure to give the treat while your dog is in the correct position—with bowed head.

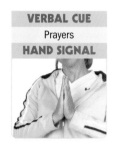

VERBAL CUE
Prayers
HAND SIGNAL

2. Now practice on a chair. Have your dog put his paws up, cue him with "prayers," and position a treat below his forearms. Using the "**bow**" cue (page 164) may help him get the idea to lower his forequarters.

3. As he improves, have your dog wait a few seconds before releasing the treat from your closed fist. In its final stage, when you point to the chair and say "prayers," your dog should assume the praying position until released.

WHAT TO EXPECT: Always offer the reward low, near your dog's chest, as rewarding from above would encourage peeking in anticipation. Dogs usually take a few weeks of squirming before they begin to understand trick.

PREREQUISITES
Paws on my arm (page 198)
Helpful: Take a bow (page 164)

TROUBLESHOOTING
MY DOG DROPS ONE PAW OFF THE CHAIR WHEN I OFFER THE TREAT
Offer the treat closer to his nose, and not as low. Your arm should be coming from below.

BUILD ON IT! Be creative—teach a doggy prayer with "amen" as your release word.

TIP! Never give your dog acetaminophen (Tylenol), as it can cause serious tissue damage.

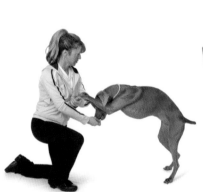

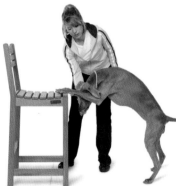

1. With his paws on your arm, offer a treat from below.

2. Transfer this behavior to a chair.

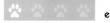
Kennel Up

TEACH IT:

When told to **kennel up**, your dog goes into his crate.

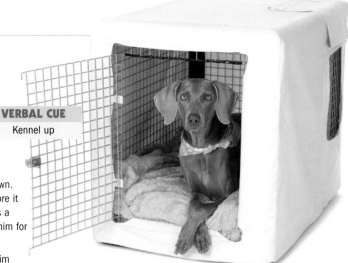

1 A crate provides a den for your dog, which instinctually feels safe. Your dog's kennel is his personal space and he deserves to be left alone while inside. Blankets and a cover make it cozy and comfortable.

VERBAL CUE
Kennel up

2 Allow your dog to approach a new kennel on his own. Tossing a few treats inside may entice him to explore it further. Once he is comfortable with his crate, toss a treat inside as you tell him to "kennel up." Praise him for going inside.

3 Now that he looks forward to this command, tell him to "kennel up" without tossing a treat inside. Once he goes in the crate, immediately praise him and give him a treat. Remember to give the treat while he is inside the kennel, as this is the position you wish to reinforce.

WHAT TO EXPECT: As part of his bedtime routine, your dog will look forward to kenneling up and receiving his good-night treat.

"I love my kennel. After a long day, I just curl up and think about things."

TROUBLESHOOTING

I HAVE A CRATE IN MY HOUSE AND ONE IN MY CAR. SHOULD I USE DIFFERENT VERBAL CUES FOR EACH?

Dogs are smart. They will understand that "kennel up" refers to any of their crates or boxes.

TIP! For a tasty treat, microwave hot dog slices for 3 minutes on a paper towel– covered plate. Cool before serving.

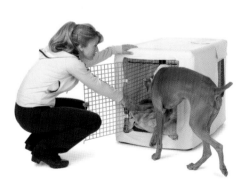

2 Toss a treat in his kennel.

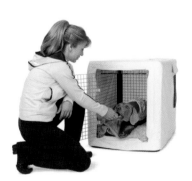

3 Give the command and then the reward.

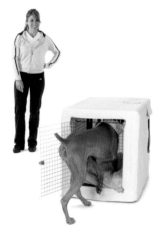

Make it a bedtime routine.

Carry My Purse

TROUBLESHOOTING

MY DOG WON'T TAKE THE PURSE OR HE IMMEDIATELY DROPS IT

If your dog is willing to take other objects, the issue may be with this particular purse. Dogs resist some textures such as metal or embellishments and smells including perfumes and cigarettes. Leather purses are a favorite.

MY DOG SOMETIMES DROPS THE PURSE AS WE WALK

Once your dog has been charged with carrying your purse, he is responsible for it until you accept it back. Sometimes, your dog will put it down for a minute to swallow or scratch—do not judge too harshly, but insist that he pick it back up.

MY DOG CHEWS THE PURSE

Hunting breeds are bred for soft mouths, while other breeds may be more prone to chewing. With any dog you're probably going to get some teeth marks on your purse eventually. Try to think of them as "character marks!"

MY DOG TRIES TO GET THE TREATS OUT OF MY PURSE HIMSELF

The treats need to be inaccessible. Try a zippered pouch.

TIP! Dogs ascertain objects that have importance to you: purse, wallet, cell phone, car keys. They will enjoy the responsibility of carrying these items.

TEACH IT:

Your little helper will carry your purse or bag as you walk.

1. Knot the straps of your purse or bag, so your dog won't become entangled. Put a handful of treats inside and close it.

VERBAL CUE
Carry

2. Hand your purse to your dog and have him **take it** (page 24).

3. Walk a few steps while telling him to "carry" and patting your leg to indicate he should come with you. If he drops the purse, do not pick it up but rather point to it and instruct him again to "take it." Your dog should only be allowed to release the purse to your hand and should not merely drop it on the floor.

4. Praise your dog as you take the purse and give him a treat from inside. When he realizes treats are inside the purse, he will be less likely to abandon it if he gets bored.

WHAT TO EXPECT: Retrieving breeds naturally enjoy walking around with things in their mouth and will likely be carrying your purse within a week.

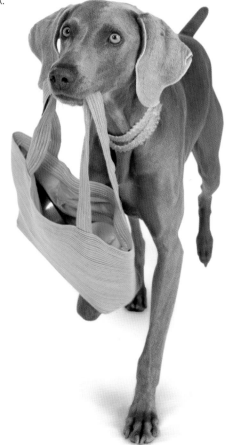

"Sometimes, I get to carry the car keys. I can make the alarm go off if I bite the keychain just right!"

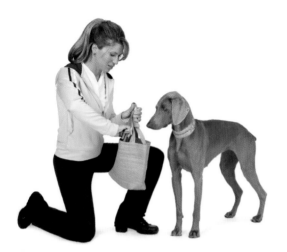

1 Put a handful of treats in your bag.

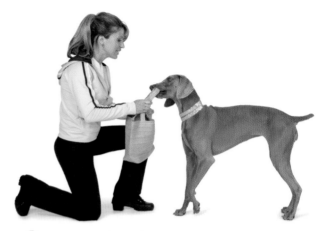

2 Have your dog "take it."

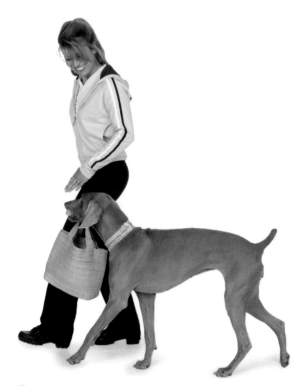

3 Pat your leg and encourage him to follow you.

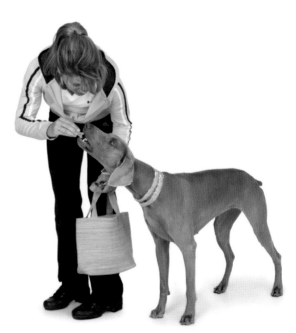

4 Pull a treat from your bag for a reward.

Tidy Up Your Toys

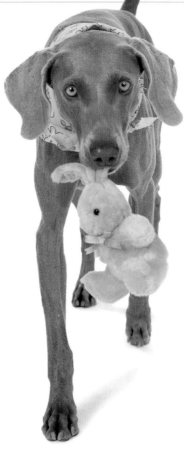

TEACH IT:

When **tidying up**, your dog opens his toy box lid, puts his toys inside, and closes the lid. First, teach the skill of putting the toys into the toy box and add to the trick later by teaching the opening and closing of the lid.

PUTTING AWAY THE TOY:

VERBAL CUE
Tidy up

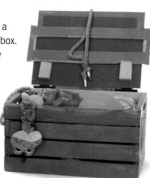

1. Scatter a few plush toys around the room and instruct your dog to **fetch** (page 24).

2. When your dog returns with a toy, offer him a treat held a few inches above the open toy box. As he opens his mouth for the treat, the toy should fall right in. Praise this success!

3. As your dog improves, stand behind the toy box with your treat tucked away. When your dog returns with a toy, point to the toy box and instruct him to **drop it** (page 26). At first, reward each successful drop in the box, and later require several toys to be deposited before rewarding.

OPENING THE LID:

1. Attach a thick, knotted rope to the toy box lid on the edge nearest the opening. The rope should be long enough so that when your dog pulls it from behind he is not hit by the lid.

2. Set your dog behind the toy box and instruct him to **pull on the rope** (page 73). At first, reward any rope pull, but as your dog improves he should be required to pull the lid completely open.

CLOSING THE LID:

1. Kneel down holding the lid straight up and encourage your dog to nose or paw it. When he does, allow the lid to fall closed and reward him. Lay a dish towel across the rim of the toy box to avoid a frightening slam.

2. Next, open the lid completely and instruct your dog to "close it." He will try a variety of actions such as nosing it, pawing it, or pulling the rope. Help him be successful by lifting the lid a few inches and encouraging him to put his nose underneath.

WHAT TO EXPECT: Once all three elements have been taught, practice them in sequence: open the lid, put away the toys, close the lid. Add this trick to your dog's daily chores, and you'll be the envy of the neighborhood!

PREREQUISITES
Pull on a rope (page 73)
Fetch (page 24)
Drop it (page 26)

TROUBLESHOOTING

MY DOG IS SOMETIMES CONFUSED AND TAKES TOYS OUT OF THE BOX!
Your dog is eager to please! "Whoops!" will alert your dog that a mistake has been made.

MY DOG WANTS TO PLAY WITH THE TOY, AND NOT DROP IT
Use less desirable toys.

"I always tidy up my plush toys first and my rubber chicken last. I don't know why, that's just what I do."

PUTTING AWAY THE TOY:

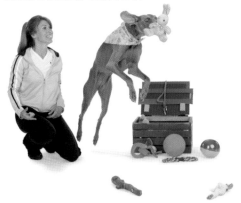

1 Have your dog fetch a toy.

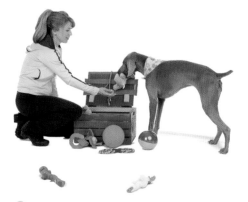

2 Offer a treat above the open toy box.

OPENING THE LID:

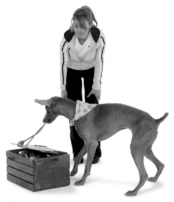

2 Instruct your dog to pull on a rope.

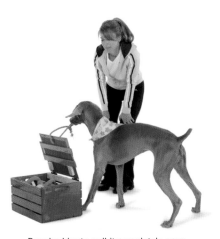

Require him to pull it completely open.

CLOSING THE LID:

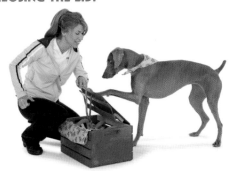

1 Hold the lid straight up and have your dog paw it closed.

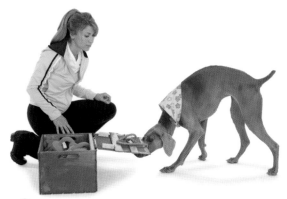

2 Open the lid completely so your dog will have to use his nose to close it.

Roll Yourself in a Blanket

TROUBLESHOOTING

MY DOG WON'T TAKE THE BLANKET
You've probably never instructed your dog to "take it" while in the down position before. Start with him standing, have him take the blanket in this position, and continue holding it while he lies down.

BUILD ON IT! Learn **say your prayers** (page 42) and **wave good-bye** (page 202) to have your dog bid good night before rolling up in his blanket.

TIP! Practice other commands while your dog holds something in his mouth: **take it, spin** or **take it, down**.

TEACH IT:

Your dog takes his blanket in his mouth and rolls over, wrapping himself up. He finishes with his head down, ready for night-night.

VERBAL CUE
Night-night

HAND SIGNAL

1. Select a blanket about two times the length of your dog. Note the direction your dog predominately rolls. If he rolls onto his left shoulder, face him and instruct him to **lie down** (page 16) on the blanket so that the majority of it is to his left. Bunch it up near his head so it will be easier for him to grab.

2. Lift the corner of the blanket and cue him to **take it** (page 24). Praise and reward him quickly when he takes the blanket in his mouth. Be sure to only reward if you take the blanket from his mouth, and not if he drops it on his own. Encourage him to stay down while being rewarded.

3. Once he is able to take the blanket and hold it, cue him to **roll over** (page 31). Dogs often release the object in their mouth when instructed to rollover. If this happens, offer neither praise nor reprimand—simply put your dog back and try again.

4. After a **rollover** is achieved with the blanket still in his mouth, instruct your dog to put his **head down** (page 56).

WHAT TO EXPECT: This trick is deceptively difficult, as your dog will need to execute each behavior perfectly in order to wrap himself up. As your dog progresses, give the "night-night" verbal cue at the beginning, and then each individual cue. In time, you will drop the individual cues.

"I have a friend next door. His name is Bear and he doesn't wear a collar and gets to sleep outside."

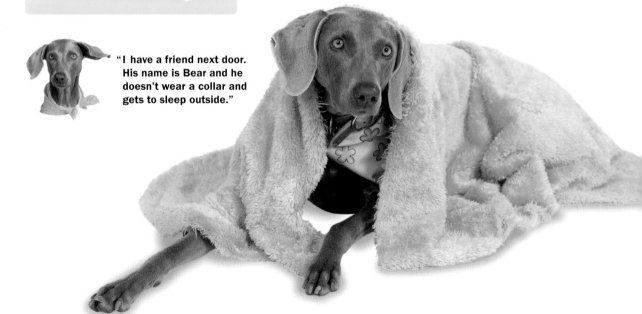

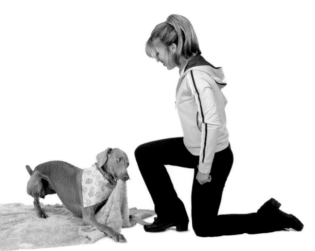

2 From a down position, instruct your dog to "take it."

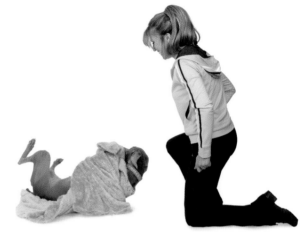

3 Have him roll over while holding the blanket.

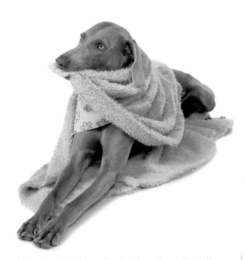

He should hold the blanket throughout the roll.

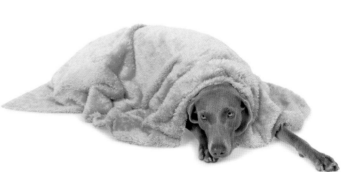

4 Head down finishes the trick.

Chapter 4

Funny Dog

Laugh and your dog laughs with you … even if you're laughing at him! One of the joys of dog cohabitation is the unabashed silliness your dog infuses into everyday life. Just as obedience is a crucial part of a successful living arrangement with a dog, so too are silly tricks an integral part of the bonding process.

If you want your dog to be well behaved and obey your commands, take an obedience class. But if you want your dog to honk a horn, play the piano, pick your pocket, and hide his head under a cushion then read this chapter! People won't be able to resist laughing as your playful pooch entertains a crowd with his antics!

Although these tricks look like pure silliness, they are based upon sound training techniques that utilize your dog's intelligence and coordination. Enjoy your funny dog!

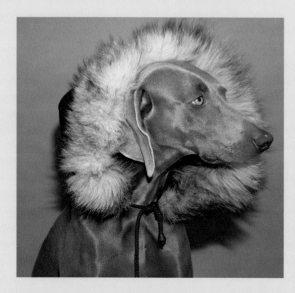

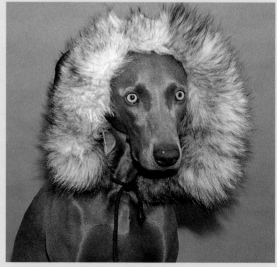

Honk a Bike Horn

TEACH IT:
Your dog bites the rubber ball of a bike horn.

1. Encourage your dog to play with a favorite squeak toy. Say "squeak!" and praise him when he produces the sound.

VERBAL CUE
Squeak!

2. This time hold the squeak toy playfully toward him as you encourage the squeak. Keep hold of the toy in one hand, and reward him with the other when he squeaks.

3. Continuing in the same session, offer the ball end of a bike horn in place of the squeak toy. Use an excited tone of voice as you encourage your dog to "squeak!" When he produces any sound, immediately give him a treat.

WHAT TO EXPECT: If your dog is a squeak toy enthusiast, he can pick up this trick in a day. It's a great trick for waking up the kids or whenever things are too quiet around the house!

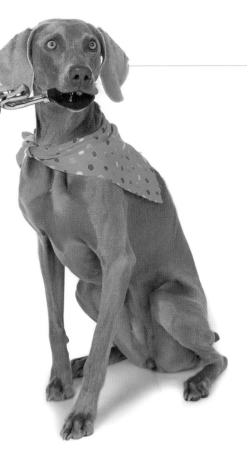

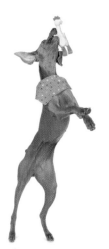

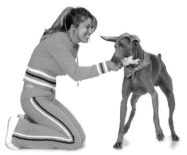

1. Say "squeak" when your dog's toy makes a sound.

2. Hold his toy and tell him to "squeak!"

TROUBLESHOOTING

MY DOG DOESN'T BITE THE HORN HARD ENOUGH TO MAKE A SOUND

The bike horn is firmer than a squeak toy, so you may have to cheat at first and squeak the horn with your thumb as your dog mouths it. He will soon learn that the sound is the desired effect.

TIP! Some human foods can be poisonous for dogs: chocolate, onions, macadamia nuts, raisins and grapes, potato peelings, tomato leaves and stems, and turkey skin.

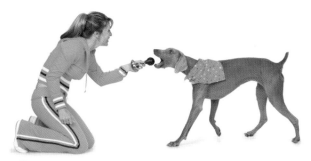

3. Use your thumb to help honk the bike horn.

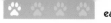
Peekaboo!

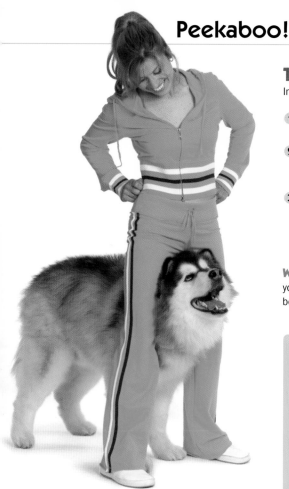

TEACH IT:

In **peekaboo**, your dog peeks out from between your legs.

1. Position yourself with your back to your dog, legs apart.

2. Reach through your legs with a treat, and lure your dog forward until he is between your legs.

3. Allow your dog to lick and nibble at the treat in your hand. Praise him with "good peekaboo," and try to keep him in this position for 10 seconds.

VERBAL CUE
Peekaboo!
HAND SIGNAL

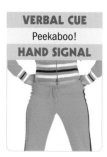

WHAT TO EXPECT: Practice ten times per day, and within a week your dog should be understanding this trick. Don't be surprised if this becomes his favorite way of getting your attention!

TROUBLESHOOTING

MY DOG BITES MY HAND AS I LET HIM NIBBLE THE TREAT
Address this issue separately. Tell your dog "easy" as you allow him to take treats. If he is too rough, bop him on the nose, and say "ouch!" to let him know he hurt you.

MY DOG IS SCARED TO BE BETWEEN MY LEGS
Your dog is putting himself in a submissive position between your legs, which requires trust. Do not force him—allow enough leash for him to back out.

MY DOG IS VERY SMALL
Kneel with your knees apart to have your dog peekaboo through that smaller space.

"Once, I peekaboo'd the delivery man and he said I should buy him dinner first."

BUILD ON IT! Once you've mastered **peekaboo**, build on this skill with **leg weave** (page 170), and **chorus line kicks** (page 176).

TIP! Save the word "no" for when your dog is naughty. Give either positive feedback or no feedback when teaching a new trick.

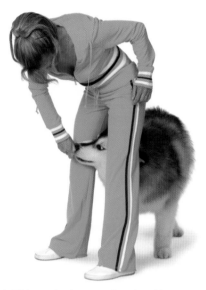

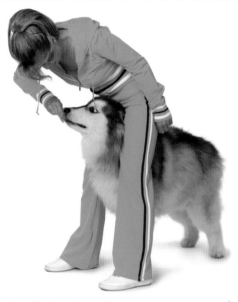

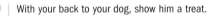

2 | With your back to your dog, show him a treat.

Lure him through your legs.

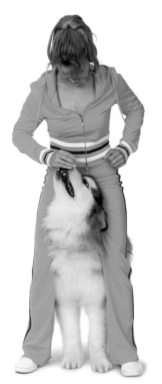

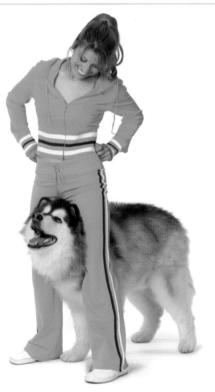

3 | Keep him in position by allowing him to nibble a treat.

Extend the length of time he stays in this position before rewarding.

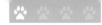

Doggy Push-ups

TEACH IT:

With paws planted, your dog does **push-ups** by alternating between lying down and standing up. Time to turn your couch potato into a hot dog—drop and give me twenty!

1 With your dog lying **down** (page 16) at your side, command him to "stand" while luring him up and forward with a treat. As soon as he rises, praise him and give him the treat.

VERBAL CUE
Down, Stand
HAND SIGNAL

2 If your dog does not respond to the food lure, use your foot to gently prod him under his belly. Reward him for standing.

3 Stand directly in front of your dog, alternating a **stand** and **down** cue to produce push-ups. Use the hand signal as well as verbal cue and for each action.

WHAT TO EXPECT: Gradually increase the number of push-up repetitions before rewarding your dog. With a solid **down** skill, your dog can be doing push-ups like a pro within a week!

PREREQUISITES
Down (page 16)

TROUBLESHOOTING

MY DOG CREEPS FORWARD EVERY TIME HE DOES A PUSH-UP

A polished push-up has little or no movement of your dog's feet. Falling back in this manner is called a "concerto" down. Practice this body movement by putting a barrier, such as an ex-pen fence, directly in front of your dog.

TIP! A treat bag at your waist offers quick access to rewards.

"Some of my favorite treats are noodles, hot dogs, string cheese, goldfish crackers, meatballs, green beans, and carrots."

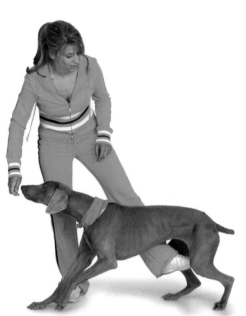

2 From a down position, lure or prod your dog to stand.

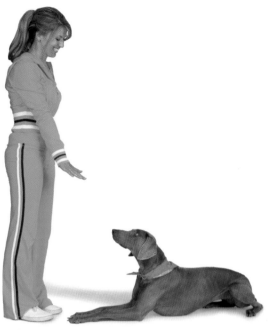

3 Once your dog is able to stand on cue, have him alternate between a down...

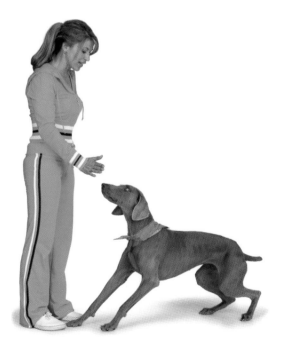

and a stand...

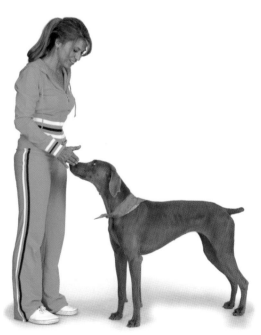

to practice doggy push-ups!

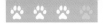

Act Ashamed

TIP! In dog trainer vernacular "cookie" means a food treat. "Do you want a cookie?"

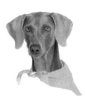

"Once, I ate a whole ham bone and then threw up. It was great."

TEACH IT:

Your dog hides his head in shame under a blanket or cushion.

1 Using a cushion that is affixed to a chair back or sofa, show your dog a treat and place it underneath, near the front. Encourage him to "get it!"

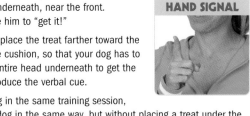

VERBAL CUE
Shame

HAND SIGNAL

2 Gradually place the treat farther toward the rear of the cushion, so that your dog has to bury his entire head underneath to get the treat. Introduce the verbal cue.

3 Continuing in the same training session, cue your dog in the same way, but without placing a treat under the cushion. As your dog sniffs around underneath, reach under the cushion from the rear, and give your dog a treat. As he improves, hold the treat in your fist for a second, instructing him to "wait, wait" before releasing it.

4 Have your dog hold his head under the cushion for a few seconds before reaching down and giving him the treat, releasing it under the cushion.

WHAT TO EXPECT: It is especially important in this trick to reward your dog while he is in the correct position. Rewarding him any place other than under the cushion will cause him to develop a habit of pulling his head out early to check for his treat. It is also preferable that you stand behind the chair, so as not to tempt your dog to pull his head out to look at you.

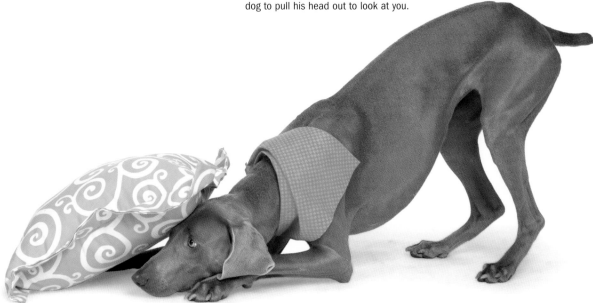

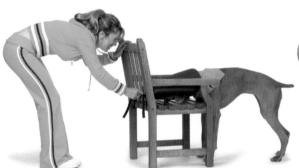

1 Place a treat under the cushion.

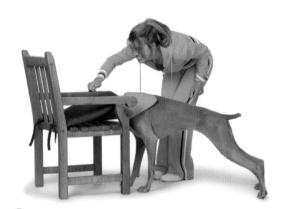

2 Place the treat farther toward the rear of the cushion.

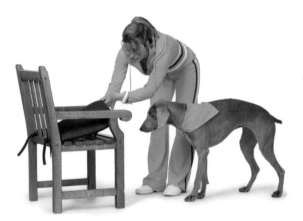

3 As your dog sniffs, reward him from behind the chair.

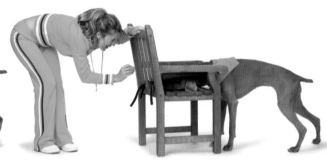

4 Have your dog wait for his reward.

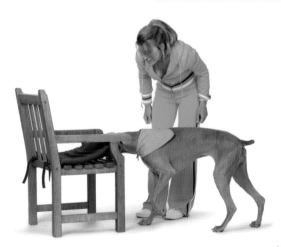

Your dog can now act ashamed on cue!

Limp

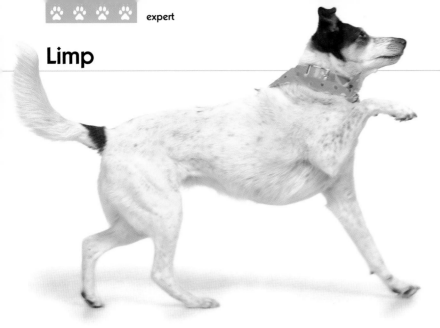

TROUBLESHOOTING

I'VE SEEN MY DOG LIMP WHEN I'VE DRESSED HIM IN A SHOE. CAN I USE THAT?

Absolutely! If you can elicit the behavior, associate it with the verbal cue "good limp!" As he improves, substitute the shoe with something smaller such as a baby's sock or tape.

WHEN DO I TRANSITION FROM USING THE LEASH TO USING THE SLING?

Switching tactics can often speed progress. Try a few repetitions with the leash, then one with the sling, then one suspending his wrist with your hand.

BUILD ON IT! Once you've mastered **limp**, learn **crawl** (page 144) and **play dead** (page 32) to act out doggy's dramatic death scene.

TIP! Dogs usually have a dominant side. Which paw does your dog prefer to raise in a **shake**? Work with this paw in his **limp**.

TEACH IT:

When performing **limp**, your dog raises his front paw while hopping on the other three. This pitiable performance can garner a free hot dog or maybe even a hot date!

1. Stand facing your leashed dog and loop the free end of the leash under his front wrist, suspending it in the air.

2. Encourage your dog to come toward you, saying "come on boy, limp." Praise and reward even one step with his free front leg. Allow your dog to rest between attempts.

3. Lighten your grip on the leash and use quick jerks rather than sustained force to encourage your dog's wrist up. Have him walk a few steps now before rewarding.

4. Fashion a sling out of fabric and loop it through your dog's collar so that it suspends his wrist. Smart dogs will figure out that they can lower their head to get out of this mess, so keep your dog's attention high as you lure him forward with a treat. You want your dog to be successful, so only ask him to do a distance he can achieve.

VERBAL CUE
Limp
HAND SIGNAL

WHAT TO EXPECT: This trick is physically as well as mentally tiring for your dog. It takes concentration for him to remember to keep the one paw lifted. As in every case where you are physically manipulating your dog, do so gently and reassuringly so as not to intimidate him. This trick can take months to master.

"I like staying in hotels. I get to drink from the ice bucket and sleep on the bed!"

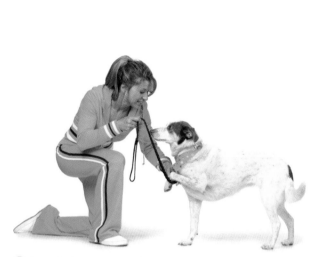

1 Loop the leash under his front paw.

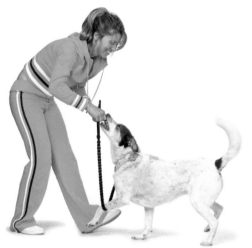

2 Reward a step with his free front paw.

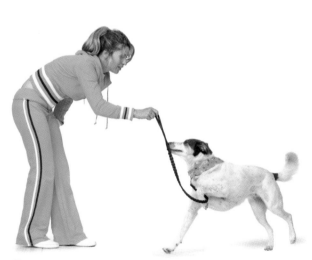

3 Use quick jerks to remind your dog to keep his paw lifted.

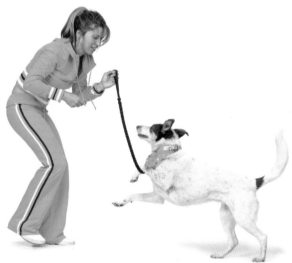

4 Have your dog limp several steps before rewarding.

Pickpocket Pooch

TROUBLESHOOTING

WHEN I HOLD THE TREAT IN MY RIGHT HAND AT THE GROUND, MY DOG GOES FOR THAT HAND INSTEAD OF MY TAILBONE
Use a treat bag at your waist or hold the treat in your mouth for easy access.

MY DOG IS TOO SMALL TO REACH MY TAILBONE ON HIS HIND LEGS
Small dogs can actually be the cutest ones for this trick. Instead of merely pushing your rear, they can learn to bounce off it with all four paws!

TIP! Have a conversation with your dog. He can understand the tone of your voice and your body language.

TEACH IT:

As you bend over to (presumably) pick up your hat, your dog swipes a kerchief from your pocket and sends you sprawling.

1 With your back to your dog, bend over with legs apart and knees bent. Hold a treat in your left hand at your tailbone. Encourage your dog to rise up and take the treat by saying "pocket, get it!"

VERBAL CUE
Pocket

2 Once your dog is performing consistently, bend over and reach with your right hand toward the ground, while still offering the treat with your left at your tailbone.

3 This time, hold the treat in your right hand instead of your left. When your dog places his paws on your tailbone, roll forward in a summersault and offer the treat in a backward motion with your right hand at the end of your roll. Practice while wearing socks, and take care to not to kick your dog.

4 Add the kerchief element by placing it in your back pocket and encouraging your dog to "**take it**" (page 24).

WHAT TO EXPECT: The difficulty in this skit will be in making the performance believable, without any noticable cues. The individual behaviors, however, can be learned within a few weeks.

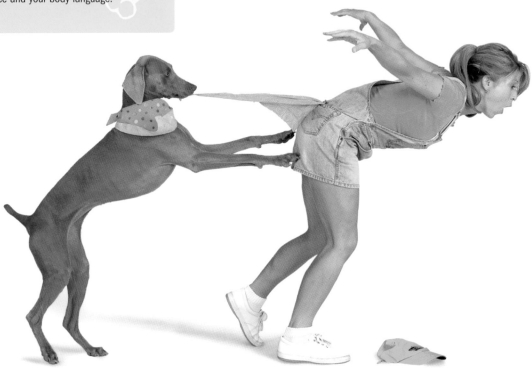

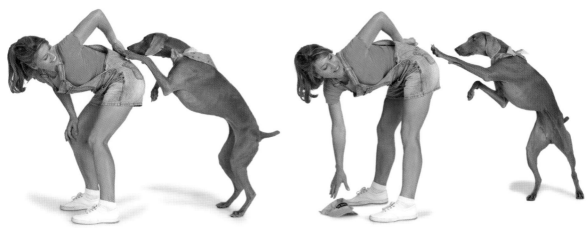

1 Bend over and offer a treat with your left hand at your tailbone.

2 Reach down with your right hand, while holding the treat with your left.

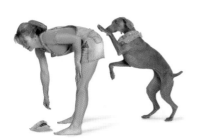 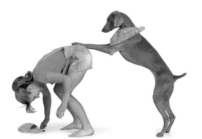 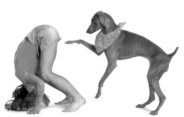

3 Hold the treat in your right hand as you reach down.

Roll forward in a summersault.

Take care to not kick your dog.

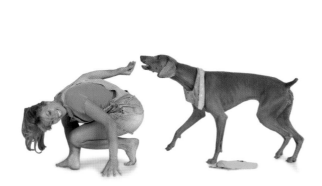 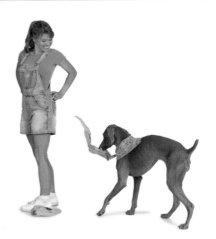

Give the treat by reaching behind with your right hand.

4 Use the "take it" cue for the kerchief in your pocket.

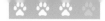

Play the Piano

TROUBLESHOOTING

MY DOG IS SCRATCHING AT THE PIANO
Do not reward scratches, but calm your dog by slowly saying "easy." Go back to tapping the back of each paw to emphasize the lifting.

MY DOG SOMETIMES MISSES THE KEYS
Use a cardboard barrier to keep your dog from putting his paws too far forward, or be quick to tap them with your finger when they land in the wrong spot.

BUILD ON IT! Learn **rollover** (page 31) to have your dog finish the song with a flourish by rolling on the keys!

TIP! If you're mad or frustrated, end the training session and try again later.

"I have my own bed. It has my name on it. Sometimes, kitty sleeps on it and gets it stinky."

TEACH IT:
Your dog will play a standard or toy piano by pounding the keys with his paws. Relaxing, isn't it?

1 Set your dog in front of a toy piano on the floor and lure him forward with a treat. As soon as he places a paw anywhere on the piano, immediately give him the treat and praise him. Be sure the treat is given while your dog is still standing on the piano.

VERBAL CUE
Music

2 The next step is to get your dog to raise and lower his paws on the piano. This will require precise timing and positioning on your part. Lure him into position, so that both paws are resting on the piano keys. Encourage him to lift one paw, by either telling him to "**shake**" (page 22) or by tapping the back side of his paw. Reward him when he puts the paw back down on the piano. His tendency will be to to put his paw down behind the piano, on the floor, so use your treat to keep his attention forward.

3 Practice one paw at a time, switching back and forth with every successful key press. Sometimes, it helps to lean your body in the opposite direction of the lifted paw. Praise should be given for placing the paw down on the piano, rather than for lifting it.

4 Stand back and let your dog play on his own! Substitute the "music" cue for "shake" and "paw."

WHAT TO EXPECT: Although this trick appears simple, the action required is a noninstinctive one. Your dog is usually rewarded for lifting his paw, rather than for lowering it.

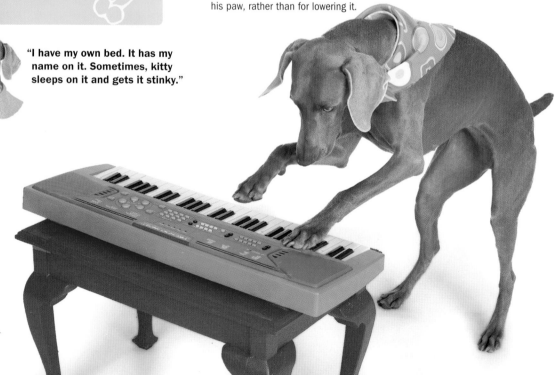

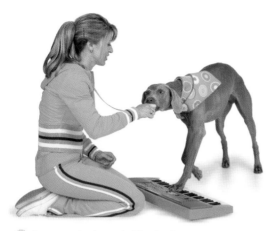

1 Lure your dog forward with a treat.

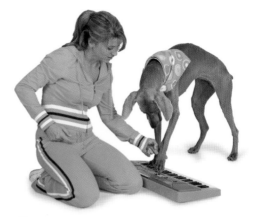

2 Cue your dog to "shake" or tap his paw.

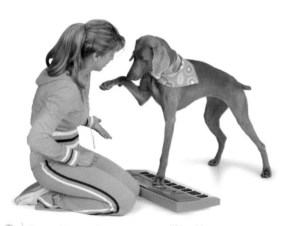

3 Lean with your dog to encourage lifting his paw.

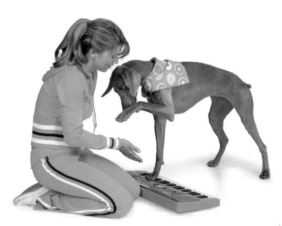

Alternate lifting each paw.

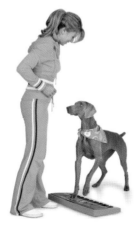

4 Stand up while continuing to cue your dog.

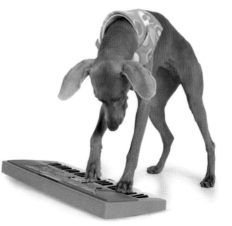

Such beautiful music!

World's Dumbest Dog

TEACH IT:

There are many variations to this trick based upon the premise that through performance art your dog responds to subtle cues making it appear that he is doing something opposite of what he has been instructed. Below are four examples:

1. "Jump, Fido, jump through the hoop of fire!" Your dog instead hides his eyes. How is this pulled off? First of all, Fido's cue for jumping through a hoop is "hup" and not "jump." Secondly, "Fido" is not your dog's name, and thirdly, your dog is responding to your subtle hand signal cueing him to **cover his eyes** (page 200). Finish this skit by saying "Fido, that cute French poodle is watching the show..." and signalling him to jump into action and through the hoop!

2. "Fido is such a well-behaved dog; he never goes in the trash." Upon turning your back to him your dog runs immediately to the wastebasket. How is this done? A treat is placed in the wastebasket, and your dog is told to stay. Upon hearing his release command, such as the word "OK" used while speaking to your audience, he will eagerly run to the trash.

3. "Where did my dog go? Has anyone seen him?" As you scan the audience your dog peeks out from between your legs. Your dog, of course, is responding to your **peekaboo** (page 52) signal.

4. "Jump through the hoop!" To your feigned embarrassment, your dog plays dead on the floor. Your dog responded to your hand signal to **play dead** (page 32).

WHAT TO EXPECT: One of the more difficult elements in this trick is getting your dog to perform a behavior behind your back, without eye contact. Dogs often will run around to look into your face. Pattern train your dog by training the exact same way every time.

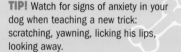

TIP! Watch for signs of anxiety in your dog when teaching a new trick: scratching, yawning, licking his lips, looking away.

TROUBLESHOOTING

MY DOG HAS TROUBLE STAYING STILL
Eye contact can be a powerful cue for your dog—make contact when you want him to *do* something, and look away when you wish him to stay.

"Sometimes, I like to pretend I don't understand anything my owner says."

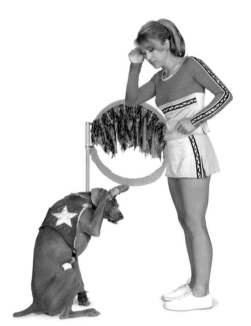

1 "Fido, jump through the flaming hoop of death!"

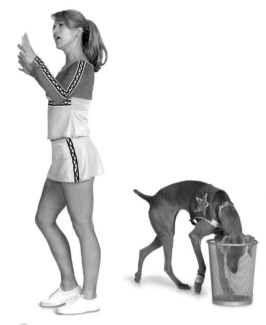

2 "Fido is so well behaved. He never gets into the trash."

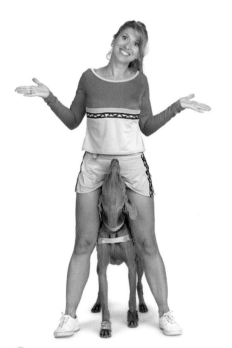

3 "I can't find my dog anywhere!"

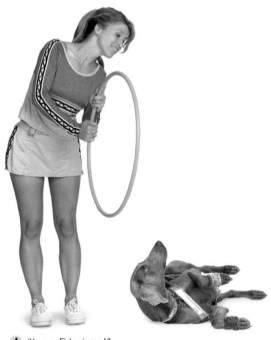

4 "Jump, Fido, jump!"

Chapter 5
Modern Conveniences

Contemporary dogs have become full-fledged family members in today's households; sleeping on beds, wearing clothing, and eating gourmet meals. Skills once required of outdoor dogs have been replaced by a more practicable set of skills geared toward today's modern living. While a dog's ability to hunt for your dinner used to be of great importance, it is now more often appreciated when a dog can find the remote control, answer the telephone, and especially bring you a cold one from the fridge!

There is something about a dog doing "people things" that we humans find endearing. When we teach a dog to respond to a cue with a natural behavior (such as fetching), we have taught him to associate a word with a particular action. When we teach a dog to execute a "people behavior," we have taught him not only the word but a complex idea involving logic and non-instinctive physical responses.

But let's be honest. The tricks in this chapter are not often taught merely to improve a dog's gray matter. They are taught for two reasons: to impress your friends and to save you a trip to the kitchen when you're thirsting for a beer!

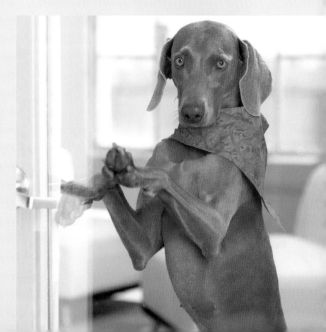

Get the Phone When It Rings

TEACH IT:

When the phone rings, your dog will pick it up from its receiver and bring it to you. With a cell phone, your dog will find it and bring it to you.

1 Set your phone on the floor and lift the receiver. Tell your dog to "**take it**" (page 24) and reward his effort.

> **VERBAL CUE**
> Rrrrrrrrrr

2 Move away from the phone and have him **fetch** (page 24) the receiver. Introduce your verbal cue by doing your best imitation of your phone's ring. Again, reward your dog for a successful retrieve.

3 Gradually move the phone back to its original spot—first moving it to a small table, then the counter, then the back of the counter. Your small dog may need a stool to reach the phone.

4 You'll now want to associate the actual phone ring with the verbal cue you were using. Use a second phone line to dial your number. When it rings, give your verbal cue and point toward the phone. Your dog may be startled for a second, but cue him each time the phone rings.

WHAT TO EXPECT: Use an old phone when learning, as dogs often drop the receiver on the floor. Keep your cell phone and treats on hand, and call your phone a few times a day. This trick involves lots of exciting things for your dog; loud noises, jumping on counters, and fetching. It's often a favorite—for both your dog and your callers!

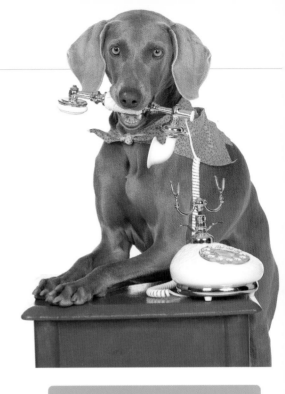

PREREQUISITES
Fetch/Take it (page 24)

TROUBLESHOOTING

MY DOG DROPS THE PHONE
Part of the problem may be the clumsy shape and slippery texture of your phone. Retro phones with a slim handle work well, or you may wish to wrap your phone with tape.

BUILD ON IT! Learn **speak** (page 30) to have your dog talk into the phone!

TIP! If you teach this trick with your cell phone, set your ringtone to an easily distinguishable, uniform ring.

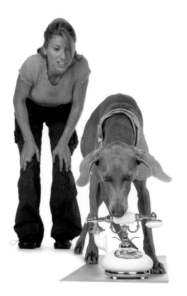

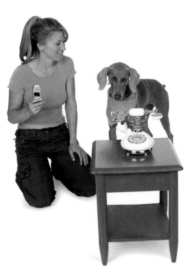

1 Have your dog take the receiver from the floor.

4 Use a second phone to teach your dog to respond to the ring.

"**When the phone rings, I pick it up and run off with it!**"

Turn Off the Light

BUILD ON IT! Once you've mastered **turn off the light**, use a similar action to learn **open/close a door** (page 70)!

TIP! Your dog should earn your praise. If you want to give him a hug, have him do a sit or a shake first.

"I have my nails trimmed twice a week. I get a cookie after."

TEACH IT:

Your dog will learn to paw a light switch on the wall, turning the lights on or off. A flat, rocker light switch is easiest, especially for flipping the switch to the up position. Small dogs may require a stool placed under the switch.

1 Hold a treat against the wall a little above the light switch and encourage your dog with "lights, get it!" Let him have the treat when he is able to reach the switch.

2 Hold the treat a little above the switch and away from the wall while tapping the switch with your other hand. Encourage your dog up again, but keep the treat clenched in your fist until he paws once or twice against the wall. Praise him and give him the treat while he is still upright.

3 Tap the switch plate while cueing your dog, then put your hands down and allow your dog to paw at the wall by himself. As he improves, challenge your dog to make a successful switch flip before he is rewarded.

4 Finally, stand across the room and send your dog by himself to kill the lights!

WHAT TO EXPECT: "Get the lights on your way out, will you?" An energetic dog can pick up the concept of scratching the wall pretty quickly, however the nuances of flipping the switch will take more time.

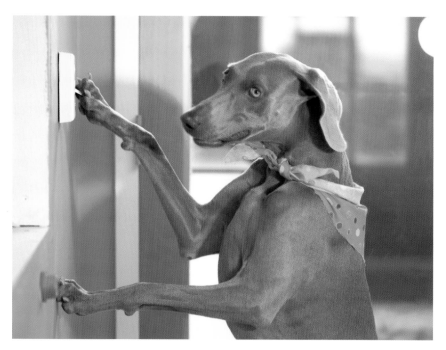

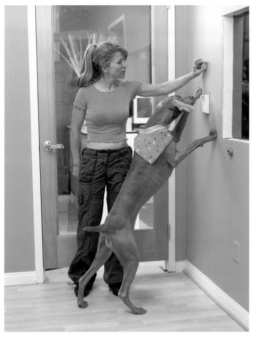

1 Hold a treat above the light switch and encourage your dog to get it.

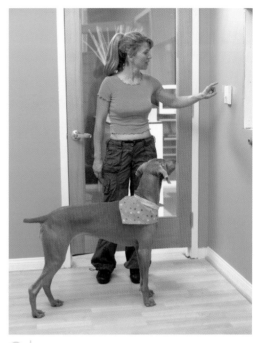

3 Tap the light switch to cue your dog to paw at it.

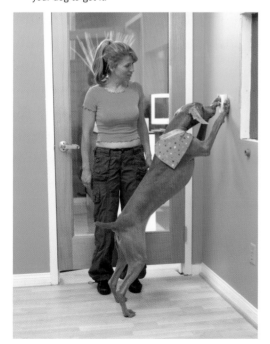

Require a successful switch flip before rewarding.

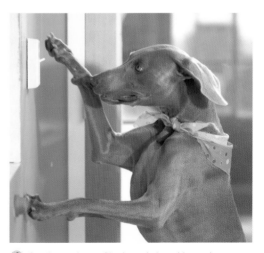

4 Send your dog to flip the switch on his own!

Open/Close a Door

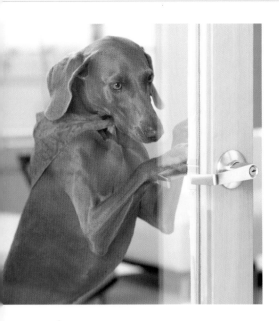

TEACH IT:

Your dog opens a door using the handle, and pushes it closed with his paws.

OPEN THE DOOR:

VERBAL CUE
Open
Close

1. Place your dog in front of an outward opening door with a lever door handle. Something desirous should be on the other side of the door, such as access to the outdoors, food treats, or a favorite toy. Have the door open a crack and encourage your dog to push his way through to get to the reward.

2. Hold the door slightly ajar, and encourage your dog to push it open. He will need to paw at it or jump on it to get it open this time. When he does, release the door, allowing it to open and giving your dog access to his reward.

3. Close the door completely and tap the door handle while encouraging your dog up. If he paws at the handle, subtly depress it and allow it to open.

4. Now that your dog understands the handle is the secret to opening doors, he will perfect his technique on his own, given enough incentive on the other side!

5. Once your dog has mastered the outward opening door, try it with an inward opening one. Tape the latch so the door opens without depressing the handle. Your dog first needs to learn to lean on the handle and walk backward. Stand on the other side of the door with a treat or toy and call to your dog while tapping on the door.

6. Remove the tape from the latch and again stand on the opposite side of the door. Keep your foot pressed against it so that if your dog depresses the handle at all, the door will open toward him. Your dog will learn to walk backward while depressing the door handle.

BUILD ON IT! Build on these skills by teaching **bring me a beer from the fridge** (page 74).

TIP! Short dogs may need a stepping stool to help them reach the door handle.

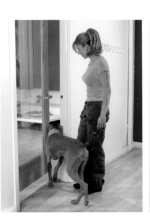

1 Have your dog push through the door crack.

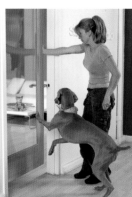

2 Hold the door ajar while your dog paws at it.

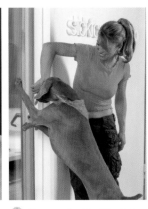

3 Depress the handle when your dog paws it.

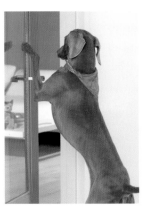

4 Give your dog incentive to open it on his own.

CLOSE THE DOOR:

7 Using a slightly ajar inward opening door, hold a treat at nose height against the door and encourage your dog to "close, get it!" When he shows interest, raise your hand higher against the door. It shouldn't take much coaxing for your dog to place his paws against the door while reaching for the treat. This will push the door closed. Immediately give your dog the treat and praise him. If he is frightened by the sound of the closing door and does not take his treat, encourage him back up on the closed door and reward him while he is in the correct position, on two paws.

8 Once your dog has the hang of this, try merely tapping the door to get him to push on it. Reward him for pushing the door closed.

9 Finally, from a distance send your dog to "close" the door. Don't be surprised if he slams it shut in his eagerness!

WHAT TO EXPECT: Door handles have baffled dogs throughout the ages. Opening a door requires both logic skills and coordination and can take a dog several weeks or more to master. Closing the door is much easier and can actually be a fun game for your dog!

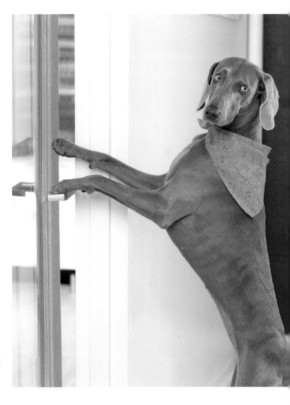

"Kitty has a little hole in the door to go through because she can't reach the handle."

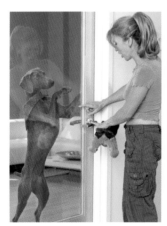

5 Try it with an inward opening door.

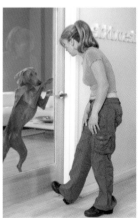

6 Press the closed door with your foot.

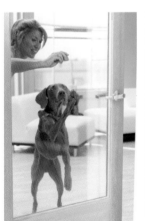

7 Hold a treat against the door.

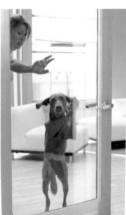

8 Tap the door.

Ring a Bell to Come Inside

TEACH IT:

Your dog noses or paws a bell on the door when he wants to go in or out.

1 Wiggle a bell on the floor and encourage your dog to "get it!" Mark the instant he touches the bell with his nose or paw by saying "good bell" and offering a treat.

VERBAL CUE
Bell

2 Hang the bell from a doorknob at a low height and encourage your dog to ring it by saying "bell, get it!" You may need to hold a treat behind the bell, and tease him with it. As soon as the bell makes a sound, praise and reward him.

3 Get your dog's leash and get him excited to go for a walk. Stop at the door with the bell, encouraging him to ring it. It may take a while, as he will be distracted by the idea of his walk. As soon as he touches the bell, immediately open the door and take him for a walk. In this trick, the reward is a walk instead of a treat, so be sure to introduce this concept early on.

4 As you return home from your walk, get him excited to go inside with promises of a treat or dinner. Again, have him paw at a bell hung from the door before opening it. It could take several minutes to ring the bell, so practice when you are not in a hurry.

WHAT TO EXPECT: Consistency in enforcing the bell to go in/out rule will speed up the learning process. You'll also need to be very responsive to the bells in the beginning—if you hear them ringing, rush to open the door. This method of communicating sure beats barking and scratching at the door, so try to reward his politeness with a walk as often as possible.

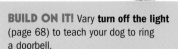

BUILD ON IT! Vary **turn off the light** (page 68) to teach your dog to ring a doorbell.

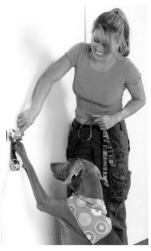

2 Encourage your dog with a treat behind the bell.

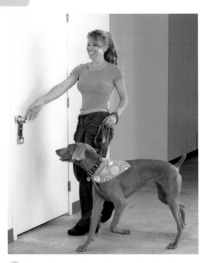

3 Reward your dog with a walk when he rings the bell.

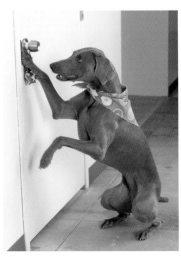

4 Have your dog ring another bell to come inside.

Pull on a Rope

TEACH IT:

Whether for opening a fence or pulling a wagon, your dog's skill at **pulling on a rope** will have endless uses.

1 Introduce your dog to **pulling on a rope** by playing tug-of-war. Pet stores sell toys and ropes for this purpose, or an old towel works well, too. Tell your dog to "tug" and wiggle the toy side to side or pull sporadically.

VERBAL CUE
Tug

2 Switch to a knotted rope. Let your dog occasionally pull it from your hands to keep his enthusiasm for the game.

3 Tie the end of the rope to a cardboard box and let him drag it around. As this is not as self-rewarding as the tugging game, be sure to praise and reward your dog for his efforts.

4 Use this newfound skill to have your dog pull a wagon with your groceries, pull open doors, or pull a rope to ring a bell. With a little imagination, your buddy will be the envy of the neighborhood!

WHAT TO EXPECT: Bull breeds and terriers are naturals for this trick, but all dogs love a good pull now and then. The more this exercise feels like a game, the faster your dog will catch on. Play daily and within a week your dog could be pulling his weight!

TROUBLESHOOTING

I HEARD PLAYING TUG-OF-WAR WITH YOUR DOG CAUSES AGGRESSION

Tug is a competitive game that results in a winner and a loser. While harmless for most dogs, aggressive dogs may interpret victory as further proof of their dominance. Enforce the rules of the game: *you* decide when the game starts and stops, the game ends with your dog relinquishing the toy, and aggression is strictly prohibited.

BUILD ON IT! Once you've mastered **pull on a rope**, your dog can open his toy box and **tidy up your toys** (page 46)!

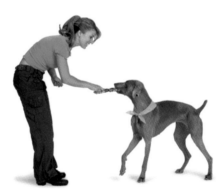

1 Play tug-of-war with your dog.

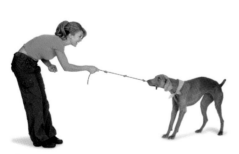

2 Use a knotted rope for this game.

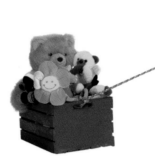

4 Attach the rope to items.

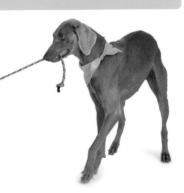

Bring Me a Beer from the Fridge

TROUBLESHOOTING

MY FLOOR IS GETTING SCRATCHED UP!
Lightweight dogs and tile floors are a slippery combination as your dog pulls the dish towel. Improve his traction with a doormat, or use a longer rope on the door handle to increase his angle of leverage.

MY DOG IS BROWSING IN THE FRIDGE WHEN GETTING MY BEER!
Nothing is free, and that just might be the price you have to pay for the luxury of beer delivery!

TEACH IT:
In this useful trick, your dog opens the refrigerator door, fetches a beer, and returns to close the door.

OPEN THE REFRIGERATOR:

VERBAL CUE
Get me a beer

1 Practice **pull on a rope** (page 73) with a dish towel. Tie the dish towel to the refrigerator handle. With the fridge door slightly ajar, instruct your dog to pull the dish towel. All four paws should remain on the floor while your dog pulls—to protect your door as well as to keep him from pushing against himself. Make it more challenging by closing the fridge door completely.

GET THE BEER:

1 Empty a beer can.

2 Play **fetch** (page 24) with the empty can to get your dog accustomed to carrying it. As many dogs are reluctant to hold metal in their mouths, a foam can insulator may help.

3 Place the beer can on a low shelf in an open, uncluttered refrigerator and have your dog **fetch** it. Reward him with a treat tastier than anything he may find in the fridge.

CLOSE THE REFRIGERATOR:

1 Cue your dog to **close the door** (page 71) while tapping the front of the open refrigerator door.

WHAT TO EXPECT: Once your dog is comfortable with all three steps, start to phase out the individual commands and use "get me a beer" to represent the entire series. Now that your dog knows the secret of the refrigerator, however, you may have to install a padlock!

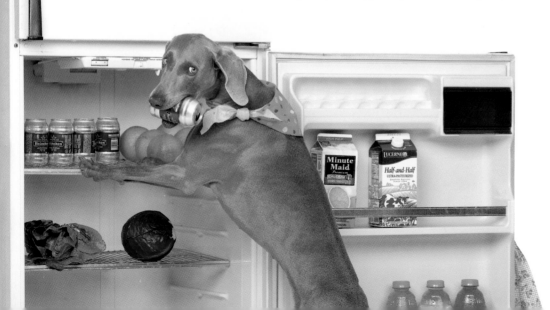

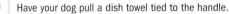

"Dad loves this trick!"

OPEN THE REFRIGERATOR:

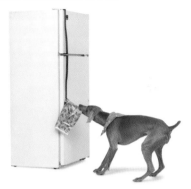

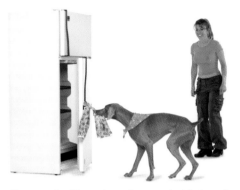

1 Have your dog pull a dish towel tied to the handle.

His paws should remain on the ground while he pulls.

GET THE BEER:

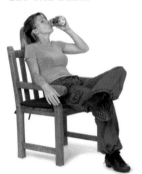

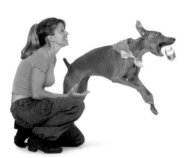

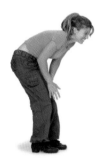

1 Empty a beer can.

2 Play fetch with the empty can.

A foam can insulator will make it easier to carry.

CLOSE THE REFRIGERATOR:

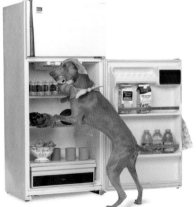

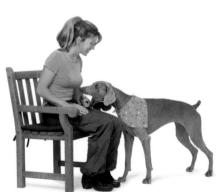

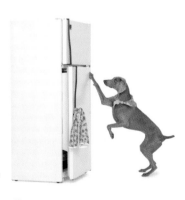

3 Fetch the can from the fridge.

Reward him for the fetch.

1 Have him return to close the door.

Mail Carrier

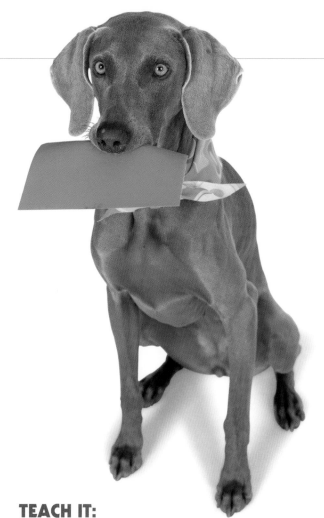

PREREQUISITES
Take it (page 24)
Give (page 26)

TROUBLESHOOTING

MY DOG DROPPED THE NOTE AND CAN'T PICK IT UP

Folding the note will make it easier to pick up.

MY DOG ENDS UP AT THE RECIPIENT, BUT WITHOUT THE NOTE!

The recipient should encourage the dog to go back and find it. "Where is it? What happened? Go get it!"

MY DOG USED TO DO THIS TRICK EASILY, BUT NOW HAS LOST INTEREST

Has he stopped receiving treats? Once learned, you need not treat every time, but at least one out of three times will keep his motivation high. You can also put the note along with a treat in a plastic baggie for him to deliver. That way the recipient can easily tip the courier!

TIP! Train your dog to deliver his charge and then run back to you for his treat!

"When I delivered the baseball, I made the umpire chase me around the field for it!"

TEACH IT:

Your dog will learn the names of family members and deliver a note to the specified recipient. When it's too important for priority mail, send it by puppy mail!

1. Have a friend or family member stand on the opposite side of an empty environment with some treats in their pocket.

2. Hand your dog a note and instruct him to "**take it**" (page 24). Point toward your intended mail recipient and tell your dog his or her name.

3. The recipient should encourage your dog to come.

4. Once close, the mail recipient should instruct your dog to "**give**" (page 26) and trade a treat for the note.

> **VERBAL CUE**
> Take it to [person's name].

WHAT TO EXPECT: Dogs remember people's names the same way we do—through repetition. Use names around your dog, and he will soon be able to identify all family members—even the cat!

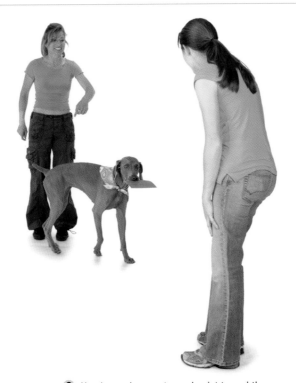

2 Hand your dog a note, and point toward the intended recipient.

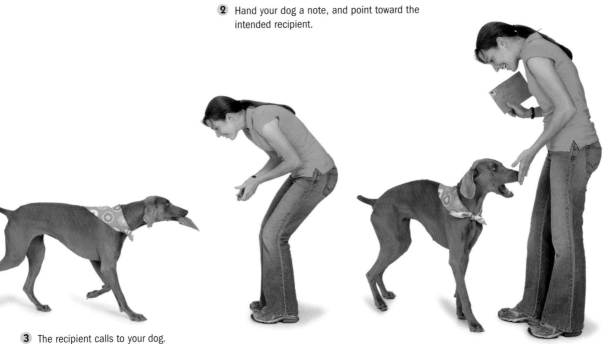

3 The recipient calls to your dog.

4 Your dog gets a treat for his delivery.

Find the Car Keys/Remote

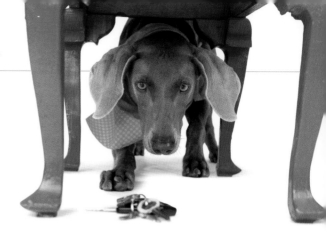

TROUBLESHOOTING

MUST I KEEP THE TREAT POUCH PERMANENTLY ON MY KEY CHAIN?
You can phase it out over time, but an object with a distinct scent will be easier for your dog to find. Rubber or leather key chains can do the trick.

TIP! Dogs see limited color. They cannot differentiate between red, orange, yellow, and green, but can tell those colors apart from blue, indigo, and violet. They perceive less detail than humans, but their night vision and sensitivity to movement is better than ours.

"I help find the kitty when she's lost."

TEACH IT:

Your dog will locate and retrieve your missing items. What a useful trick!

KEYS:

VERBAL CUE
Keys, find it
Remote, find it

1. Attach a small change purse filled with treats to your key chain. Toss the keys playfully and tell your dog "keys, **fetch**" (page 24). When he returns with the keys, open the pouch and reward him with a treat from inside. As he cannot open the pouch on his own, he will learn to bring it hurriedly to you. The scent of the treats in the change purse will help your dog find your keys.

2. Next, hide the keys farther away, or in the next room. Make a game of it and help your dog search room to room. The next time you lose your keys, you'll be glad you put in the effort of teaching this trick!

REMOTE:

1. A hard plastic remote is not an object that most dogs take readily in their mouths, so you may wish to wrap it in masking tape during the learning process. Show the remote to your dog and tell your dog "remote, **take it**" (page 24). Praise him and exchange it for a treat.

2. Set it on the coffee table, point to it, and say "remote, **fetch**."

3. Set this trick in a realistic context. Sit in your armchair and set the remote in a commonly found spot. Have your dog fetch it and bring it to your chair. Your guests will be amazed by this useful trick!

WHAT TO EXPECT: Although teaching your dog to retrieve a named object is not a complicated process, the challenge in this trick will be keeping your dog's motivation high when the object you are having him seek is not a toy or treat. Be sure to give lots of praise and rewards during the learning process, and within a month your dog can be finding and retrieving your lost items!

STEPS:

KEYS:

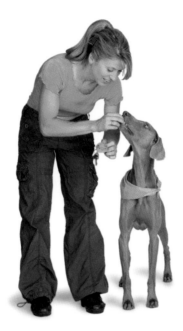

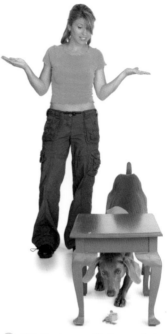

1 Fill a key chain pouch with treats. Reward your dog for fetching it.

2 Hide the keys and help your dog search for them.

REMOTE:

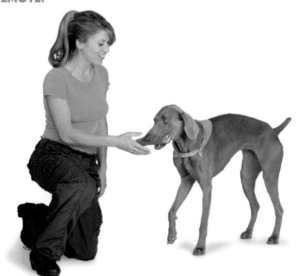

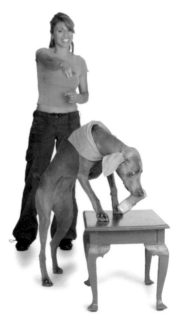

1 Wrap the remote in tape and have your dog take it in his mouth.

2 Set the remote on a coffee table and have your dog fetch it from a distance.

Push a Shopping Cart

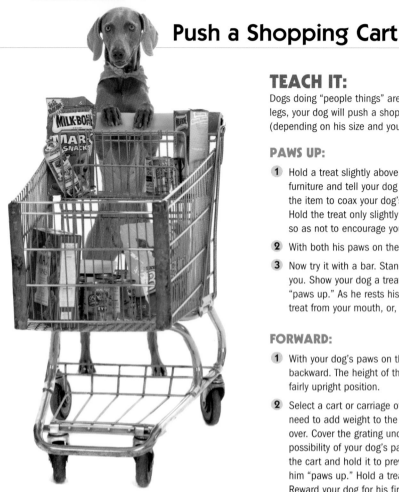

TEACH IT:

Dogs doing "people things" are always entertaining. Standing on his hind legs, your dog will push a shopping cart, baby carriage, or toy lawn mower (depending on his size and your household chores!).

PAWS UP:

VERBAL CUE
Paws up
Forward

1 Hold a treat slightly above a sturdy piece of furniture and tell your dog "paws up." Pat the item to coax your dog's front feet onto it. Hold the treat only slightly behind its edge, so as not to encourage your dog to jump on top or over it.

2 With both his paws on the item, allow your dog to take the treat.

3 Now try it with a bar. Stand facing your dog, holding the bar between you. Show your dog a treat held in your mouth, and instruct him "paws up." As he rests his paws on the bar, allow him to take the treat from your mouth, or, if you prefer, spit it into his mouth.

FORWARD:

1 With your dog's paws on the bar, tell him "forward" as you walk backward. The height of the bar should cause your dog to be in a fairly upright position.

2 Select a cart or carriage of appropriate height for your dog. You may need to add weight to the basket to prevent your dog from tipping it over. Cover the grating under the handle with a towel to prevent the possibility of your dog's paws getting stuck in it. Stand to the side of the cart and hold it to prevent it from rolling. Tap the handle and tell him "paws up." Hold a treat in front of him and coax him "forward." Reward your dog for his first steps, and remember to always give the reward while the dog is still in the correct position, standing up.

3 Stand at the opposite end of the cart and use a treat near your dog's nose to lure him forward. Over time, lighten your grasp on the cart and soon your dog will be shopping on his own!

WHAT TO EXPECT: A grassy surface works well for this trick, as it will slow the cart down. Keep control of the cart during the learning process, as a slip could cause significant setbacks.

TROUBLESHOOTING

MY DOG KEEPS LOWERING HIS FRONT PAWS TO THE GROUND
Use your treat as the "carrot," holding it just inches from his nose as he walks forward.

BUILD ON IT! Adapt **tidy up your toys** (page 46) to have your dog fill his cart with groceries before wheeling off!

PAWS UP:

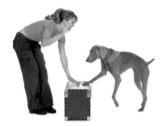

1 Hold a treat high as you tell your dog "paws up."

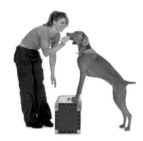

2 Give the treat while both of your dog's paw are up.

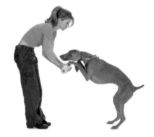

3 Transition to having your dog lift his paws to a bar.

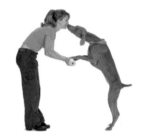

Allow your dog to take a treat from your mouth.

FORWARD:

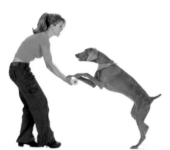

1 Walk backward.

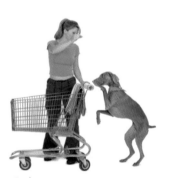

2 Lure your dog's paws up.

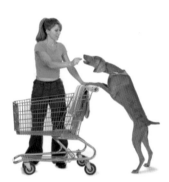

Move the treat to coax him forward.

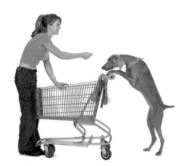

3 Stand on the opposite side of the cart.

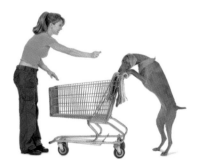

Over time, lighten your grasp.

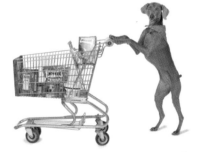

Soon he'll be shopping on his own!

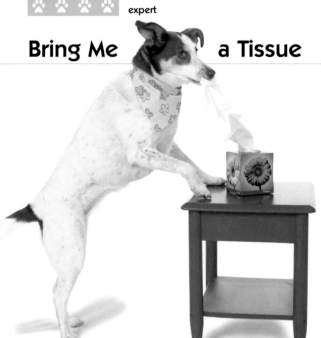

expert

Bring Me a Tissue

TEACH IT:

Your sneeze is your dog's cue to fetch a tissue from its box for you. When you have finished with it, your dog can even toss it into the waste can.

FETCHING THE TISSUE:

1 Secure a box of tissues to a low table or the floor using duct tape. Wiggle the exposed tissue and tell your dog to "**take it**" (page 24).

2 Move a little away from the tissue box. Point to it and say "Achoo! **Fetch**!" Encourage your dog along the way, then instruct him to "**give**" (page 26) or trade him a treat for the tissue.

3 Try it while sitting in a chair. Try moving the tissue box to different places. Phase out the extraneous commands until your only cue is "Achoo!" Hold the treat in your hand as you do the hand signal to keep your dog focused.

DISPOSING OF THE TISSUE:

4 While sitting in a chair with a wastebasket at your side, crumple the tissue and hand it to your dog, saying "**take it**, throw it away."

5 Point to the wastebasket with a treat in your pointing hand, while repeating "throw it away." As your dog comes closer to sniff the treat, instruct him to "**drop it**" (page 26). When he drops the tissue, drop your treat into the wastebasket and let him get it. By giving the treat in the wastebasket, he will be eager to stick his nose in there, increasing his chances of dropping the tissue in the correct place.

6 As your dog improves, move the wastebasket farther away.

WHAT TO EXPECT: Fetching the tissue is usually easier to teach than disposing of it. Although the basics may be taught in a few weeks, performing the trick with only one verbal cue will be more difficult. Just think of how impressed your guests will be when you sneeze and your dog comes running in with a tissue!

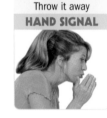

VERBAL CUE
Achoo!
Throw it away

HAND SIGNAL

PREREQUISITES
Fetch/Take It (page 24)
Drop it/Give (page 26)

TROUBLESHOOTING

WHILE I WAS OUT, MY DOG EMPTIED THE ENTIRE TISSUE BOX!
Some dogs find this incredibly fun! Be thankful your playful pooch hasn't discovered the toilet paper roll!

MY DOG DROPS THE TISSUE
Go back and work on **fetch** (page 24). If your dog drops the fetch item, do not pick it up, but rather encourage him to bring it the rest of the way to you.

THE TISSUE STICKS TO MY DOG'S LIPS WHEN HE TRIES TO THROW IT AWAY
The tighter you ball up the tissue, the easier it will be for your dog to release it. You can also slip a rock into the tissue ball.

MY DOG TAKES THE TISSUE FROM THE BOX DIRECTLY TO THE WASTE CAN
Make sure he sees your treat as you do your sneeze hand signal. Hold eye contact draw him in to you.

FETCHING THE TISSUE:

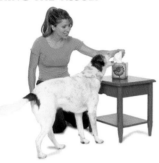

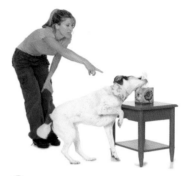

1   Tape the tissue box to a table and have your dog "take it."   **2**   Point to the box and say "achoo! Fetch!"

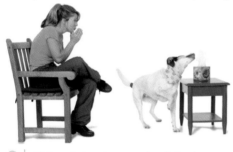

3   Sit in a chair and use your hand signal.   Trade your dog a treat for the tissue.

DISPOSING OF THE TISSUE:

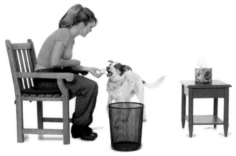

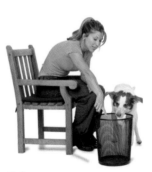

4   Hand the crumpled tissue to your dog.   **5**   With a treat in your hand, point to the wastebasket.

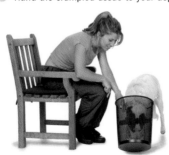

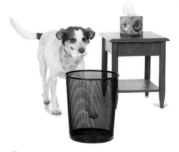

Drop the treat in the wastebasket.   **6**   Move the wastebasket farther away.

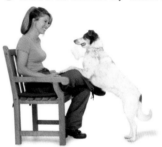

Chapter 6

Let's Play a Game!

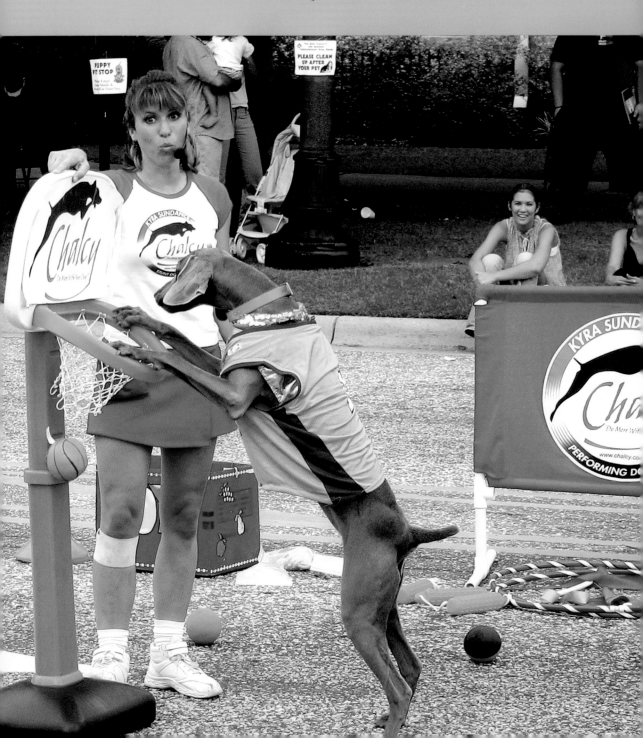

G-o-a-l!

The crowd goes wild as your canine athlete scores one for the team! Nicknamed the Flying Fido, your dog will shoot, dunk, catch, and block his way into the heart of your entire neighborhood once he learns how to participate in your games. He's sure to be the first one picked on your team!

What do friends do on their weekends off? They play sports! Whether it's flag football in the park or foosball in the game room, sporting competition has always been a shared bond between best buds. Now, with these tricks, your canine companion can be included in your games.

Whether he's partial to the pigskin, a fan of the free throw, or has a super slap shot, your dog can learn the rules to these popular sports and play alongside you.

Playing a game with your dog builds communication skills as well as establishes rules that will penetrate throughout your relationship. Think of yourself as a coach while teaching these tricks. Use energy and motivation in equal parts with discipline and authority. The game should be a reward in itself, and your dog will be required to follow rules in order to get this reward. Be fair, be honest, and be patient. Every big-league star started in the pee-wees and your dog will start there, too.

Let's go outside and play!

Soccer

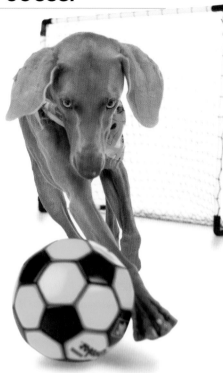

TEACH IT:

Sports fans are sure to get a kick out of your superstar dog as he goes for the goal by rolling a **soccer** ball into a net.

1. A treat ball toy sold in pet stores is a hollow plastic ball with a hole that, when rolled, randomly releases treats. Fill it with kibble or goldfish crackers and allow your dog a few days to play with it on his own. It will likely become a favorite toy.

> **VERBAL CUE**
> Soccer

2. Point to an empty treat ball and tell your dog "soccer!" When he rolls the ball a few feet, toss a treat near the ball for him to find.

3. Gradually require longer roll times before rewarding, and switch to rewarding from your hand instead of tossing the treat.

4. Substitute a soccer ball, giving the same verbal cue and rewarding for a short roll. Gradually build up the distance.

5. Is your dog ready to try a goal? Set a distinct line in front of the net, such as the edge of a concrete surface next to a grass field. Run excitedly with your dog and encourage him to push the ball past this line. When he does, reward him immediately.

WHAT TO EXPECT: Dogs often learn to roll the treat ball on their own quickly. There can be some confusion when transitioning to the soccer ball requiring you to switch back and forth between the two. Practice daily and in a few weeks your dog can be on his way to the World Cup!

"Here's my favorite game: chasing bumper. Here's my other favorite game: chasing frisbee."

TROUBLESHOOTING

MY DOG SKINNED HIS NOSE!

With a brand new treat ball, or a very enthusiastic roller, a dog can develop scratches on his nose. Check his nose often and inspect the ball for snags.

MY DOG PAWS AT THE SOCCER BALL INSTEAD OF ROLLING IT

Your dog is frustrated and not understanding what you want. Go back to using the treat ball, but put only one kibble in it. Your dog will hear that there is something in it, but the kibble will take a longer time to come out. Reward your dog for rolling it with treats from your hand.

TIP! Freeze some chicken broth into ice cubes for a hot weather treat.

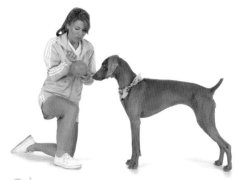

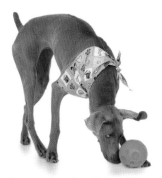

1 | Fill a treat ball with kibble.

Let your dog play with it on his own.

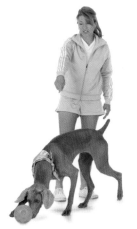

2 Using an empty treat ball, toss the treat to your dog when he rolls the ball.

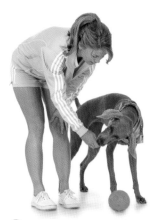

3 Transition to rewarding from your hand.

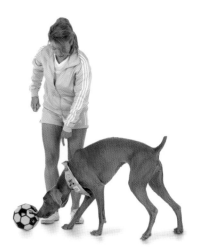

4 Reward a short roll with a soccer ball.

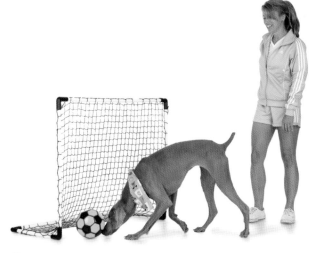

5 Set a distinct goal line for your dog to cross.

Football

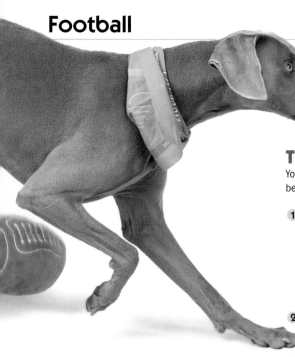

TEACH IT:

Your dog will play both center and receiver as he hikes the **football** between his legs and then goes long for the catch.

1 Drop a plush football in front of your dog and tell him to "hike!" He won't know what you want, but your excited tone will encourage him to try different things: picking it up, dropping it, throwing it in the air, barking, bringing it to you, pawing it. When he touches it with his paw, mark that instant by exclaiming "good!" and quickly giving him a treat.

VERBAL CUE
Hike

2 Gradually require him to paw harder at the football in order to earn the treat. Continue to mark the instant he produced the desired behavior by exclaiming "good hike!"

3 Chain several behaviors together: have him **drop** (page 26) the football, **bow** (page 164), "hike," and then **catch** (page 92) after you throw it. Your dog's possessiveness of his toy may lead him automatically to cover it with his paws when doing his bow. If not, your dog will learn in time that "hike" comes after "bow" and will cover the ball in preparation for this next cue.

WHAT TO EXPECT: This trick can be frustrating for you and your dog at the beginning, as he needs to experiment with different behaviors until he stumbles upon the desired one. Your timing in marking the instant he gives the behavior is crucial. Have patience; with consistent training your dog could become a gridiron great!

PREREQUISITES
Drop it (page 26)
Take a bow (page 164)
Hockey goalie (page 92)

TROUBLESHOOTING

MY DOG'S HIKE LACKS FORCE
Some dogs tend to push the football through their legs rather than fling it. Withhold treats until your dog gets frustrated and flings it hard. Then give him a jackpot—a whole handful of treats!

TIP! Dog training is a lesson in self control—*your* self control.

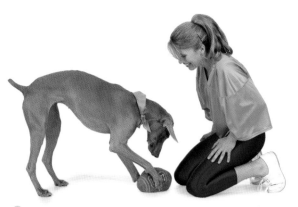 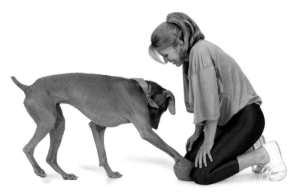

1 Encourage your dog to play with a football and reward him for touching it with his paw.

2 Require your dog to paw at it harder to earn the treat.

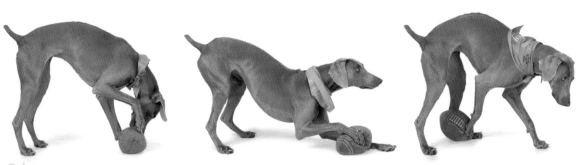

3 Play a game by having your dog drop it,   bow,   hike,

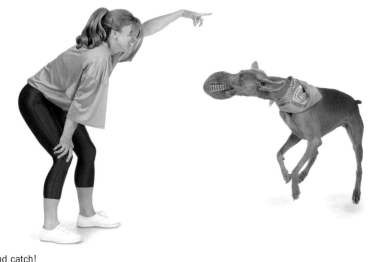

and catch!

Basketball

TROUBLESHOOTING

MY DOG'S BASKETBALL KEEPS MISSING THE NET

Your dog's initial success in making the basket is largely dependent on the timing and placement of your reward. Watch his head and hold the treat in a location that will cause the ball to fall in the net when your dog opens his mouth for the treat.

BUILD ON IT! Two nets, two dogs, and a bucket full of balls make a rousing game of dog basketball!

TIP! The more it feels like a game, the more enthusiastic learner you will have.

TEACH IT:

Your dog will slam dunk the competition when he nets the basketball. Add a second dog for competition, or challenge your friends!

1. Set the net of a toy basketball stand low enough that your dog can reach it while standing on four paws. Toss a toy basketball for him to **fetch** (page 24).

VERBAL CUE
Dunk

2. Coax him toward a treat held against the backboard while telling him to "dunk."

3. As he reaches toward the treat, command him to "**drop it**" (page 26). He should release the ball into the net as he opens his mouth for the treat.

4. At first, reward him for dropping the ball anywhere near the net. As he improves, require a successful basket before rewarding.

5. Challenge your dog further by tapping the backboard instead of holding a treat against it. As your dog progresses, the verbal cue "dunk" will come to mean the entire action of fetching the ball and dropping it in the net.

WHAT TO EXPECT: Practice this trick ten times per session, keeping the training energetic and fun. Within a few days you'll likely see some progress. Real athletes will be able to stand on their hind legs to reach a higher net. Now that's a slam dunk!

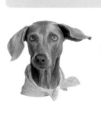

"I wear rubber boots when I do basketball halftime shows. They make me run funny and they're sticky."

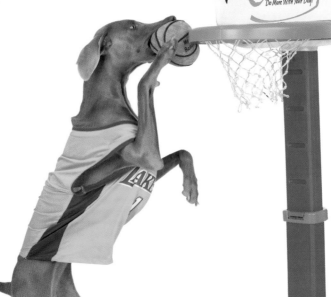

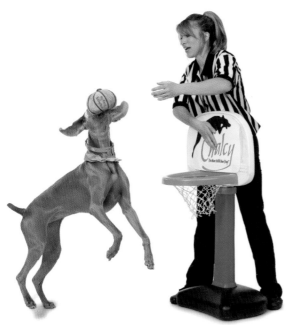

1 Toss a basketball for your dog to fetch.

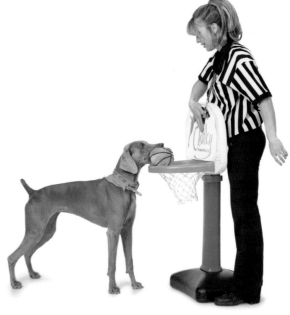

2 Coax him toward a treat held against the backboard.

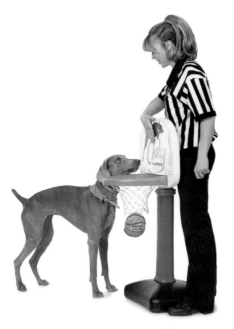

3 As he reaches for the treat, the ball should drop into the net.

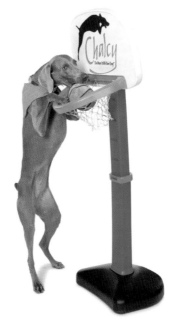

5 Soon your dog will be slam dunking on his own!

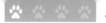

Hockey Goalie

PREREQUISITES
Target (page 145)

TROUBLESHOOTING

IS IT NORMAL FOR A DOG TO STAND THERE AND WATCH THE BALL HIT HIM ON HIS HEAD?

This sometimes happens. You probably shouldn't toss the ball directly at him, just in case he's not in a catching mood.

TIP! Tennis ball crazy? Excessive mouthing of tennis balls can cause damaging tooth wear. Rubber balls are a better alternative.

TEACH IT:

Your **hockey goalie** dog will ice the competition as he positions himself in front of the net to catch anything whacked his way!

1. Most dogs will learn to catch on their own; we are now just associating a word with that action. Select an object that is easy for your dog to catch, such as a plush toy. Play keep-away with it for a minute, then toss it to your dog and say "catch!" Praise him, repeating the cue "good catch, good catch." Treats are not used in this trick, as catching is a self-rewarding activity.

VERBAL CUE
Catch

2. Have your dog **sit** (page 15), while you back up and toss the toy to him. Vary the toys and balls, cueing "catch" each time.

3. Now it's time to place the net behind your dog and whack the ball to him with a hockey stick. You don't want to hurt your dog, so use soft, easy to catch balls that are too large to be swallowed.

4. After catching your shot, your dog will probably engage in a victory lap around the yard. The trick now is to get him to position himself back in front of the net. With a cleverly placed **target** object (page 145) in the center of the net, cue him to touch the target. As soon as he does, yell "catch" and whack the ball to him, which serves as his reward.

WHAT TO EXPECT: Ball-crazy dogs will play hockey goalie for hours. The real work could very well be in honing your skills as a shooter!

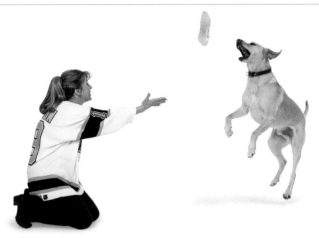

1. Toss a plush toy for your dog and say, "catch!"

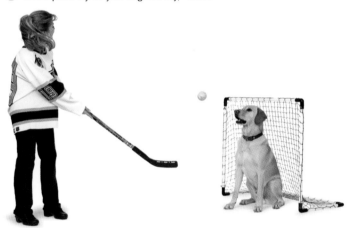

3. Incorporate the net and stick and hit a soft ball toward your dog.

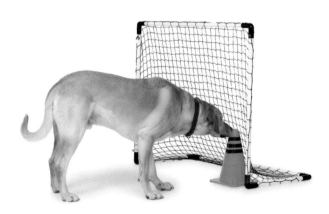

4. Touching a target will bring him back in front of the net.

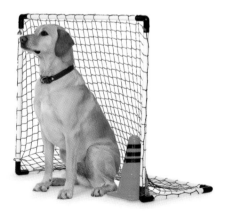

Reward your dog with another ball!

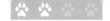

Hide-and-Seek

TROUBLESHOOTING

WHEN I LEAVE THE ROOM, MY DOG CHEATS AND BREAKS HIS STAY!
Check back on him periodically and return him to his original spot if he has moved. When your housemate is cooking dinner, set your dog in the kitchen so his stay can be enforced.

BUILD ON IT! Switch the game around. Learn **go hide** (page 96) to have your dog do the hiding while you seek.

TIP! This trick also helps your dog learn your name.

TEACH IT:

Your dog holds a stay while you find a hiding spot. Upon yelling a release word, he comes looking for you!

1 Hide-and-seek is a game, not an obedience drill. Make it fun for your dog with high energy and laughter! Position your dog in a **sit-stay** (page 15 and 18) and walk to the other side of the room. Call your dog to **come** (page 19) and reward him with a treat.

2 Again put your dog in a stay, and walk just outside the room. Call him enthusiastically to "find [your name]" and praise and reward him when he does.

3 Choose a more difficult hiding spot, such as behind a door. Call to him loudly when you are settled in your spot. Your dog will use his keen canine nose to sniff you out!

4 Is the game getting too easy for your dog? He can actually smell the path to your hiding spot. Make it more difficult by walking into several rooms before choosing your final spot.

WHAT TO EXPECT: This trick is a wonderful combination of fun and learning! Discipline is practiced in your dog's stays, and he gets to hone his scent-tracking abilities. Most dogs love this game and will sniff you out quicker than you can count to twenty!

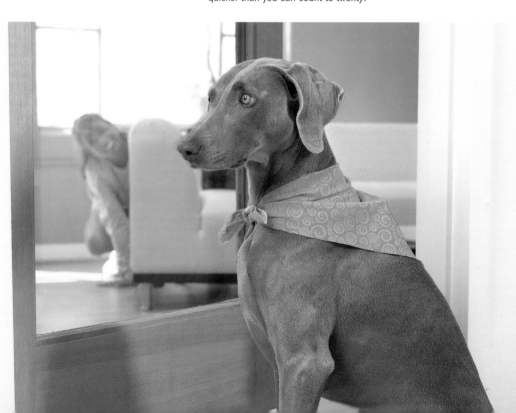

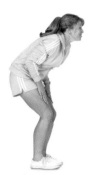 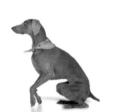 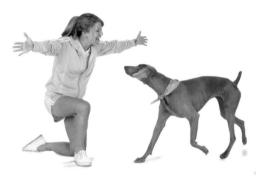

1 Position your dog in a sit-stay, and then call him to "come."

Treat this like a game, and not an obedience drill.

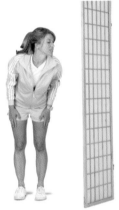 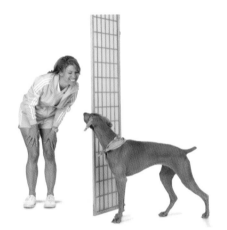

2 Hide just outside the room and call to your dog to "find [your name]!"

Praise your dog for finding you.

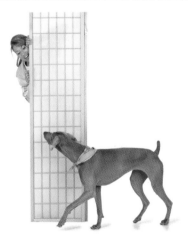

3 Choose more difficult hiding places, such as behind a door.

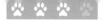
Go Hide

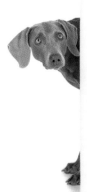
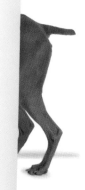

TEACH IT:

When you tell your dog to "**go hide**," he hides behind any object. A big dog trying to hide behind a skinny pole is always good for a laugh!

1 This trick is picked up easiest by toy-motivated dogs. Get your dog excited with a game of **fetch** (page 24).

VERBAL CUE
Go hide

2 Set a large object, such as an upturned picnic table, in your play area. Show your dog a treat and tell him to "go hide" as you toss it behind the table. Praise him for going behind the table, then immediately get his attention and toss his toy into the yard. The toy serves as his reward, while the treat is merely used to cause him to go to the correct place.

3 Wean off the treats as you just tell him to "go hide" and point to the table. Your dog may only go half way to the table, in which case walk toward him as you keep pointing and cueing. You may even have to walk all the way to the table to get him to go behind it Don't reward him with his toy until he is in the correct spot. The toy is his incentive, and the more he wants it, the quicker he will learn.

4 Once he is hiding behind the table, try other objects. Point to a tree or the corner of a building and have him hide there.

WHAT TO EXPECT: You may have already witnessed this behavior in your dog as he stalks prey. Toy-motivated dogs can be hiding within a few weeks. Require your dog to be well hidden before getting his reward, or he will develop a habit of peeking or inching forward.

TROUBLESHOOTING

MY DOG ISN'T INTERESTED IN TOYS

Is he interested in treats? Have him hide and then toss a treat to him. Be sure to toss the treat, rather than having him come back to you for it, as that would encourage him to come out of his hiding spot.

TIP! Remove your sunglasses. Eye contact is key to training.

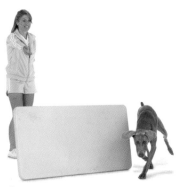

2 Toss a treat behind the table and tell your dog to "go hide."

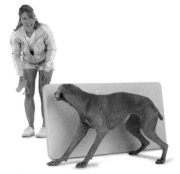

3 Wean off treats as you point to the table and say "go hide."

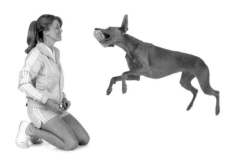

Reward your dog with a toy.

Which Hand Holds the Treat?

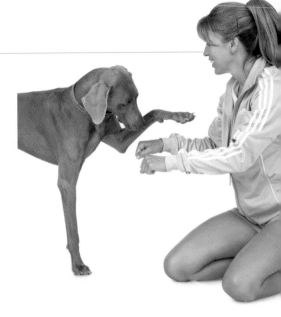

TEACH IT:

When presented with your two closed fists, your dog sniffs each and indicates **which hand holds the treat**.

1. Using a treat with a strong smell, such as hot dogs, place it slightly exposed in one of your two fists. Face your dog with your fists at his chest height. Ask him "which hand?" and encourage him to "get it!"

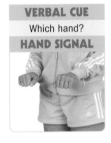

VERBAL CUE
Which hand?

HAND SIGNAL

2. When your dog shows interest in the correct hand, either by nosing it for a few seconds or pawing it, say "good!" and open your hand to allow him to take the treat. Repeat with the treat in the other hand.

3. If your dog shows interest in the wrong hand, tell him "whoops," open that hand to show him it is empty, and stop the trick. Wait 30 seconds before trying again so that there are negative consequences to his incorrect choice.

4. Increase the difficulty by covering the treat entirely with your hand, while still leaving an air hole for your dog to sniff.

5. Wait until your dog is consistently choosing the correct hand before changing his indicator requirement from nosing your fist to pawing at it. Keep your fists low to the ground. When your dog has indicated his choice with his nose, pull your other hand back and encourage him to paw at your correct hand by saying "get it!"

WHAT TO EXPECT: This trick involves two of your dog's favorite things: using his nose and getting treats! Dog's usually catch on pretty quickly, but achieving a high rate of accuracy will require your dog to calm down and take this task seriously.

TROUBLESHOOTING

I THINK MY DOG IS JUST GUESSING

Overly zealous dogs will be in such a hurry to get the treat that they paw at the first hand they see. Try holding your fists up above your dog's head so he can sniff them but not paw them. After he has sniffed both, tell him to "wait," lower your hands, and then ask "which hand?"

MY DOG SCRATCHES MY HAND

Let your dog know he hurt you by saying "ouch! Cut it out!" Gloves may be helpful until he has mastered this trick.

BUILD ON IT! Once you've mastered **which hand**, increase the difficulty by giving your dog three choices in **shell game** (page 102)!

TIP! Groom your dog often to help prevent skin disease.

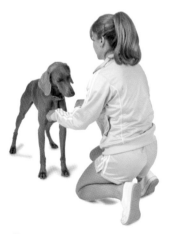

1. Present your fists to your dog and encourage him to "get it!"

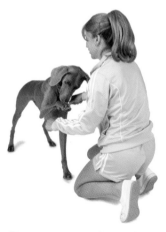

2. Reward your dog for showing interest in the correct hand.

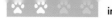
Easter Egg Hunt

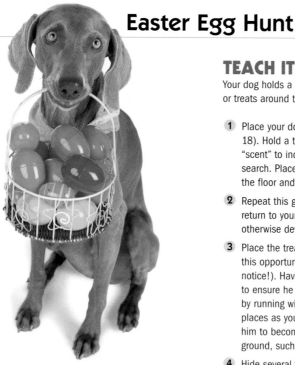

TEACH IT:

Your dog holds a sit-stay while you play Easter bunny, hiding colored eggs or treats around the house. Release your dog to find as many as he can!

1 Place your dog in a **sit-stay** (page 15 and 18). Hold a treat to his nose and tell him "scent" to indicate the scent he is to search. Place the treat a few feet away on the floor and send him to "find it!" Praise him when he does.

VERBAL CUE
Scent
Find it

2 Repeat this game again, placing the treat a little farther away. Always return to your dog before releasing him from his **stay** as he may otherwise develop a bad habit of sneaking while you are out of sight.

3 Place the treat out in the open, in the next room. Many dogs will use this opportunity to try to sneak into your room (thinking you won't notice!). Have a friend monitor your dog, or return to him frequently to ensure he stays put. If your dog seems confused, encourage him by running with him toward the treat. Increase the difficulty of hiding places as your dog improves. Monitor his success, as you don't want him to become frustrated and give up. Try hiding spots higher off the ground, such as on a coffee table or stairs.

4 Hide several treats around the house at one time, and see how many your dog can find.

5 Try this game with a colored egg or ball. Hold the ball to your dog's nose and tell him "scent." Hide it in an easy spot, and when he finds it encourage him to bring it back to you for his treat.

WHAT TO EXPECT: This is a favorite trick for dogs, as they love to use their nose and enjoy the hunt! Vegetables as hidden treats offer a low-calorie alternative and are just as much fun. You can expect your pooch to catch on to the concept within a week.

"I looooove this game! I know all the hiding places and can find all the treats before my owner is finished making my dinner."

PREREQUISITES
Stay (page 18)

TROUBLESHOOTING

MY DOG GIVES UP TOO QUICKLY
The object is not to outwit your dog, but to make him successful. Progress slowly so your dog builds confidence in his ability. Over time, he will enjoy greater challenges. Strong smelling treats will also be easier to find.

CAN I PLAY THIS WITH EASTER EGGS?
Absolutely! Show your dog an egg as you tell him to "scent," and send him on his way. Be warned—the eggs may be eaten before they make it into the basket!

TIP! Consistently hide eight treats before dinnertime. Your dog will come to inherently know the number of treats to be found, and you will have several minutes of peace while preparing his dinner.

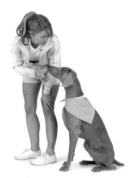 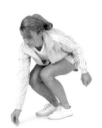 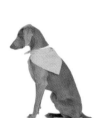 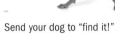

1 Hold a treat to your dog's nose and tell him "scent."

Place the treat a few feet away.

Send your dog to "find it!"

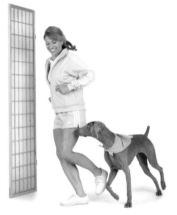 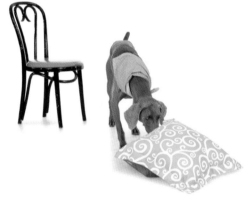

3 Place the treat in the next room and run with him to find it.

4 Hide several treats and see how many your dog can find.

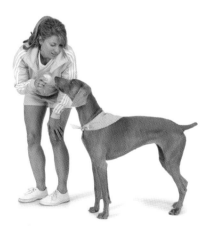 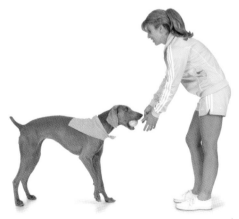

5 Hide a ball instead of a treat.

Reward your dog for bringing the ball back.

Ring Toss

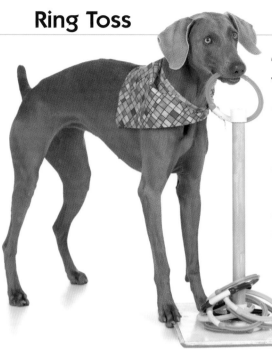

TEACH IT:

Your dog maneuvers rings onto an upright pole.

1. Introduce your dog to the pole by tapping it and saying "**target**" (page 145). Practice the **target** skill a few times by rewarding your dog each time he touches the pole.

| VERBAL CUE |
| Ring it |

2. Plastic diving rings can be purchased at pool supply stores. Hand your dog a ring and have him **take it** (page 24). You'll want him to hold the north side of the ring, with it circling his chin.

3. With the ring in his mouth, cue your dog to touch the **target**.

4. Once your dog is able to touch the target while holding the ring in his mouth, offer his treat near the top of the pole and instruct him to **drop it** (page 26). Reward your dog for dropping the ring anywhere near the pole.

5. As your dog improves, reward him only for dropping the ring onto the pole. Tap the pole to focus his attention and lure his head forward with a treat until the bottom of the ring catches on the pole. Tell him to "drop it" and immediately praise him and give him the treat if the ring lands on the pole. If the ring misses the pole, say "whoops!" and try again.

6. Once your dog has mastered this skill, ask him to pick up the ring from the ground or from another pole instead of from your hand. He might pick it up holding the south side of the ring, which will probably cause him to miss the pole. Through trial and error he will discover on his own that he needs to hold the north side. If he does pick up the south side, he will learn to relax his grip, allowing the ring to swivel downward. Dogs are very smart!

WHAT TO EXPECT: Although this trick looks incredibly difficult, dogs often pick it up easier than you would expect! Practice only about five times per session in the beginning, as it can be frustrating for your dog. Remember to end with a successful attempt.

PREREQUISITES

Take it (page 24)
Target (page 145)
Drop it (page 26)

TROUBLESHOOTING

MY DOG GETS THE RING ON THE POLE, BUT IMMEDIATELY TAKES IT OFF AGAIN

Your dog is excited and forgetting to let go of the ring. When he gets the ring partially on the pole, hold your finger to the top of the pole to prevent him from removing the ring. He'll quickly get the idea.

BUILD ON IT! This skill can be translated into dropping a coin into a piggy bank or maneuvering the ring onto your extended arm.

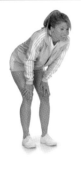
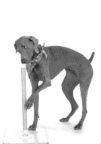
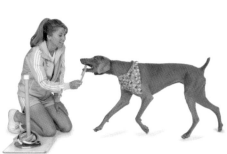
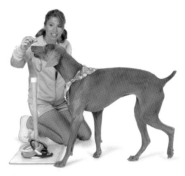

1 Identify the pole as the target.

2 Hand your dog the ring by its north side.

4 Offer a treat near the top of the pole.

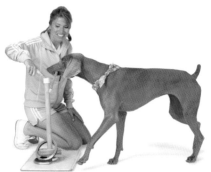
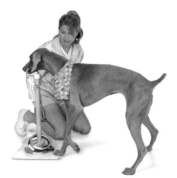

5 Focus his attention to the pole until the bottom of the ring catches.

Instruct him to "drop it."

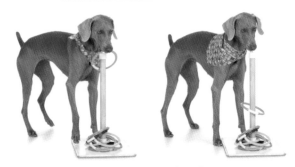
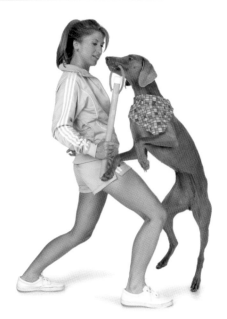

Reward your dog for getting the ring on the pole.

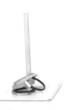
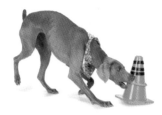

6 Have your dog pick up the ring from another pole.

Vary the trick by holding the pole yourself.

Shell Game

TROUBLESHOOTING

CAN I USE CUPS INSTEAD OF FLOWER POTS?

Clay flower pots work well because their weight and shape prevent them from overturning too easily. Convenient scent holes encourage your dog to sniff the top instead of the base, reducing sliding across the table—cups can overturn or smash when pawed.

TIP! Monitor the amount of treats you give and deduct it from your dog's dinner.

TEACH IT:

In this classic con game, a pea is placed beneath one of three shells. After the con man quickly shuffles the shells, the audience bets on which one hides the pea. No sleight of hand can trick your nosy dog as he sniffs out the pea!

1 Start with just one clay flower pot on the floor. Rub the inside with a treat to give it lots of scent. Let your dog watch as you place a treat on the floor and cover it with the pot. Encourage him to "**find it**!" (page 98.) When he noses or paws the pot, praise him and lift it to reward him with the treat.

2 After your dog catches on, which shouldn't take long, hold the pot in place and keep encouraging him until he paws at it. Tap his wrist or use the word "**shake**" (page 23) to give him the idea to use his paw. Reward any paw contact by lifting the pot. Strive for a soft paw indication and do not allow your dog to tip the pot over by himself.

3 Add two more pots and mark the scented one so you don't forget! In a soft voice, tell your dog to "find it!" Tap the first pot to direct his nose there, and then the second, and third. If your dog paws at an incorrect pot, do not lift it, but rather say "whoops" and encourage him to keep looking. Use the pitch of your voice to calm your dog as he diligently sniffs each pot and to excite him when he shows interest in the correct one. If your dog loses interest, quickly lift and set back down the correct pot to show him the treat. Hold the pots firmly in place while your dog sniffs to prevent him from pawing one over by himself.

4 Place the pots on a low table for an added challenge. Place a treat under one and shift them all around. Your dog should indicate the correct cup with a soft paw.

WHAT TO EXPECT: Scenting tricks can be mentally tiring for your dog. Be gentle with your negative feedback. Only practice a few times per session and end with a successful attempt.

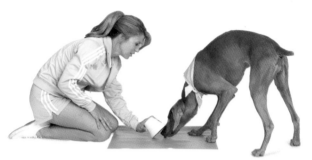

1 Place a treat under a pot. Lift it when your dog noses it.

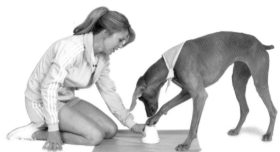

2 Hold the pot in place until your dog paws at it.

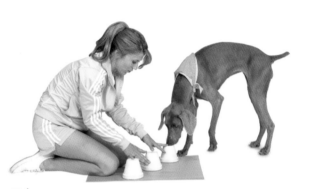

3 Add two more pots. Hold them in place and direct your dog to sniff each.

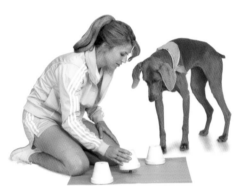

Quickly show him the treat if he loses interest.

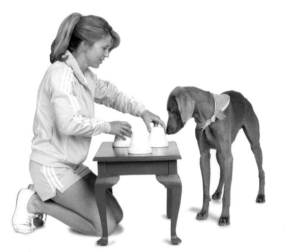

4 Shuffle the pots on a low table.

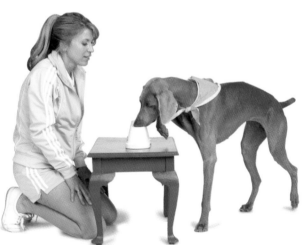

Your dog should indicate the correct pot with a soft paw.

Dog on Point

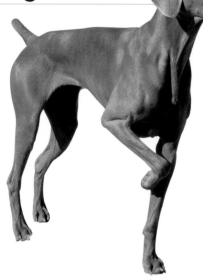

TEACH IT:

Pointing prey is an instinctive behavior that you may have already observed in your dog. When on point, the dog's stance is frozen with body outstretched and tense, erect tail, alert ears, and foreleg lifted with foot curled slightly into their body.

1 Rather than training this trick during your normal training session, be observant of a time when your dog exhibits this behavior naturally. If you catch him staring intently at a bird, tense your body and crouch down to further engage his pack hunting instinct. In a low voice, build his intensity by saying "what is it? Are you gonna get it?" Move in close but do not attempt to go ahead of him, as this can cause him to break. Your goal is to keep him in this intense position as long as possible.

VERBAL CUE
Point

2 Train outdoors as it is a more stimulating environment. Toss around your dog's favorite ball to build his drive. Hold him by his collar and toss the ball several yards. Use as few words as possible so as not to distract him while you get him to **stay** (page 18) while standing.

3 Walk over to the ball while keeping your eyes on your dog, enforcing his stay. Bat the ball around to pique his interest. Release your dog with "OK!" to pounce on his prey. Because his release will come at random times, he will learn to tense his body and point in anticipation of the pounce.

4 As your dog improves at holding point, encourage good form by stroking the underside of his tail and tapping his paw.

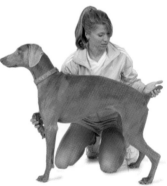

WHAT TO EXPECT: Sporting dogs and high prey-drive dogs will take to this trick easiest, while gentle dogs may never show the intensity required to attain a rigid point.

PREREQUISITES
Helpful: Stay (page 18)

TROUBLESHOOTING

WON'T THIS ENCOURAGE MY DOG TO CHASE SMALL ANIMALS?
Pointing and chasing are two different things. Seeking and pointing are self-rewarding activities, and the chase need not be involved.

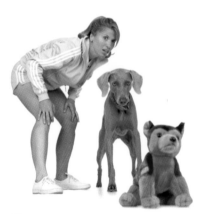

1 Notice when your dog naturally stares and build his intensity.

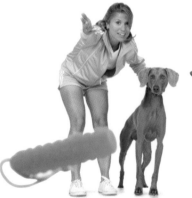

2 Hold your dog's collar as you toss his toy.

4 Encourage good form.

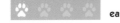
3-2-1 Let's Go!

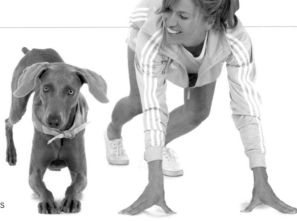

TEACH IT:

You and your dog hold your mark as you count down from three. On the cue of "let's go!" you race off together shouting and barking and causing household havoc!

1 When your dog is in a happy and excited mood, hold him by his collar at your left side. Crouch down as if you are about to sprint and in a suspense-building drawn-out tone say "threeeeee..."

> **VERBAL CUE**
> 3-2-1 let's go!

2 Your dog will likely be very excited and try to break away. Hold his collar and tell him to **stay** (page 18). Use a coaching tone, as opposed to a commanding tone, as you want to keep him excited for the release.

3 Continue on with "twooooo.... oooooone..." and then release his collar shouting "let's go!" and sprinting away from him. No treats are necessary as this is a self-rewarding game.

4 Require your dog to stay during the "3-2-1" without holding his collar. If he breaks, stop the game and order him back. Start over with "3."

WHAT TO EXPECT: The intelligent (and conniving) animals that they are, dogs often learn the pattern of "3-2-1 ..." and take off a half second before your cue! It's a good exercise in discipline to enforce the stay.

> **PREREQUISITES**
> Stay (page 18)

> **TROUBLESHOOTING**
>
> **MY DOG GETS CRAZY EXCITED!**
> Dogs can go bonkers with this game and can hurt themselves or you with their wild abandon so be smart about your surroundings. Use this game to amp up your dog up before an agility competition or to encourage more exercise.

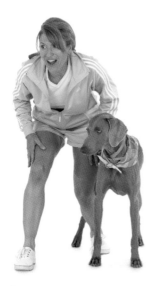
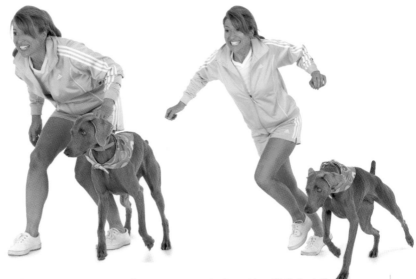

4 Require your dog to stay as you say "threeeeee..."

"twooooo.... oooooone..."

and release him with "let's go!"

Chapter 7

Jumping and Catching

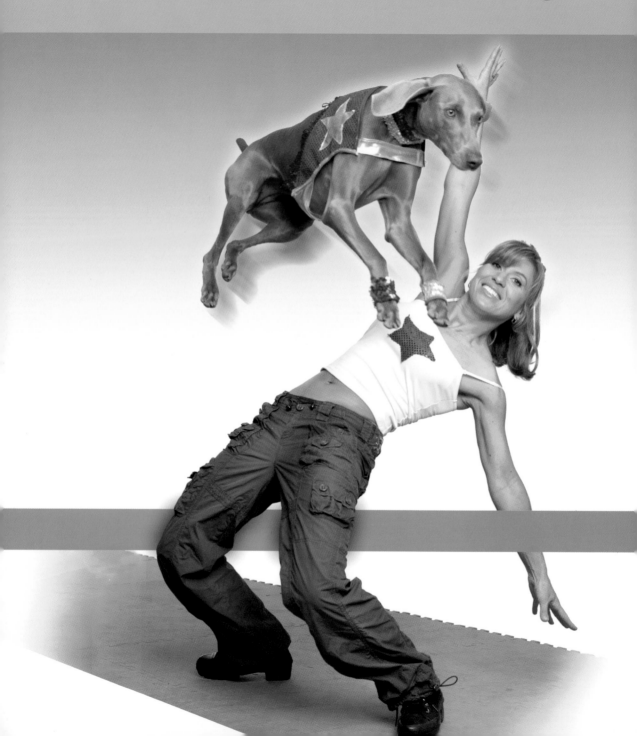

Teamwork

Teamwork is the name of the game as you and your partner perform synchronized jumps and catches. You'll learn to trust and read each other as you work collaboratively to execute a stunt. The rewards are in the journey and the successes are measured in the smiles, barks, and tail wags of you and your best bud.

Dogs love to jump—it's an exhilarating and self-rewarding behavior. Jumping and catching tricks are impressive to the onlooker as they showcase your dogs' speed, grace, coordination, and athleticism. A jumping dog is a happy dog, and people can't help being inspired by his zest for life!

Jumping is also a strenuous behavior, and a painful one if the dog is not at a high fitness level or has health problems or injuries. Keep a close eye toward signs of discomfort, and remember to stretch, warm-up, and cool-down your dog. Do not encourage him to jump higher than he can achieve with moderate effort, and control his form so that he jumps and lands straight and close to horizontally.

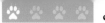
Jump Over a Bar

TEACH IT:

Your dog will learn to **jump over a bar**.

1   Set up a bar jump or create a homemade version out of two chairs and a broomstick. For safety reasons, the bar should release if hit. Set the bar to a low height: 3"–6" (7.5–15 cm) for small dogs and 12"–18" (30.5–46 cm) for medium-sized dogs.

VERBAL CUE

Hup or jump

2   With your dog on a lead, run with him toward the jump. Give an enthusiastic "hup!" as you jump over the bar with him and praise him for his success. A treat may be given, however most dog enjoy the jump on its own. If your dog is reluctant, lower the bar to the ground and walk over it with him. Avoid pulling him over the jump, and give him plenty of encouragement.

3   As your dog's confidence improves, gradually raise the bar. Try sending your dog over the jump from different positions. Put your dog in a **stay** (page 18), and call him from the opposite side of the jump. Or stand on the side of the jump and wave him over. Have your dog do figure 8's over the jump: jump forward, circle the left side and back to you, jump forward, circle the right side and back to you.

WHAT TO EXPECT: Most dogs enjoy jumping and will take to it easily if given positive feedback. Within a few days, your dog can be a jumper!

TROUBLESHOOTING

MY DOG TRIPPED ON THE BAR AND IS NOW SCARED OF IT

Much of his memory of this episode will be determined by your reaction. Encourage your dog to "walk it off" and in the future make sure the bar has a release and the ground is not slippery. Instead of a leash that can become tangled, use a tab—a short lightweight rope.

BUILD ON IT! Build on this skill to teach **jump over my back** (page 110).

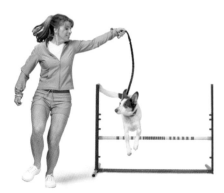

2   Run with your leashed dog over the jump.

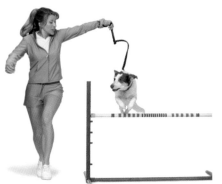

3   Gradually raise the height of the bar.

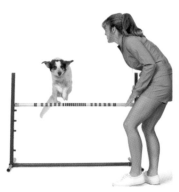

Stand on the opposite side of the jump and call your dog over.

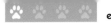
Jump Over My Knee

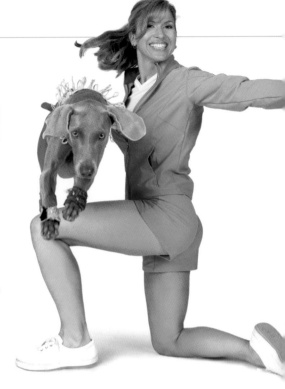

TEACH IT:

As you kneel on the floor, your dog jumps over your raised thigh.

1 With your dog on your left, kneel on the ground with your right leg outstretched. Rest your foot against a wall. Lure your dog over your leg with a treat. Tell him "hup!" as he moves over your leg. If he attempts to go under your leg, move your leg lower.

> **VERBAL CUE**
> Hup

2 Raise your leg up a little higher. Your dog may be tempted to cross near your ankle as that is the lowest spot, so keep your treat close to your body to tempt him in that direction. An enthusiastic voice will stimulate a higher jump!

3 Kneel with your thigh horizontal and your knee against the wall. If your dog tries to go under your leg, lure him slowly so that he first places his front paws on your thigh. Allow him to nibble the treat from this position, then move the treat farther away from him and use an enthusiastic "hup!" to coax him to jump the rest of the way.

4 Move away from the wall and use a sweeping motion of your right arm to signal your dog to jump over your knee.

WHAT TO EXPECT: This is a fun trick for your dog, and one that can be achieved by most dogs. Practice when your dog is full of energy and he should get the hang of it in a week or two!

> **BUILD ON IT!** Jumping over your knee is the first step in learning **jump into my arms** (page 112)!

> **TIP!** Have your dog **circle behind you** (page 166) in preparation for a second jump.

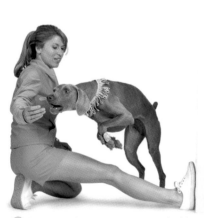

1 Lure your dog over your outstretched leg.

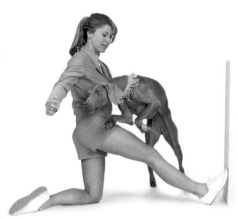

2 Raise higher and tell your dog to "hup!"

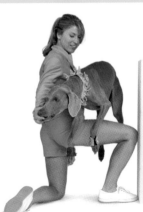

3 Kneel with your knee against the wall.

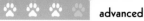
Jump Over My Back

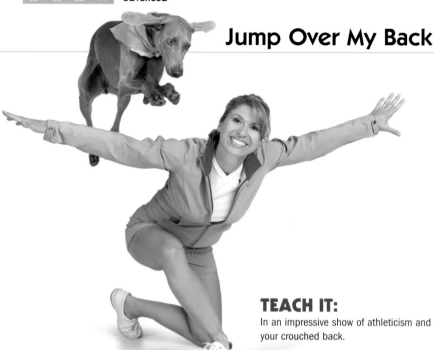

TEACH IT:

In an impressive show of athleticism and teamwork, your dog jumps over your crouched back.

1. Stand next to the upright while you have your dog **jump over a bar** (page 108). Set the bar height to about 24" (61 cm).

2. This time, crouch down next to the upright.

3. Kneel on your hands and knees under the bar and instruct your dog to jump. If he is reluctant, have a friend encourage him over. If your dog has trouble at any point learning this trick, go back to the previous step.

4. Remove the bar from jump, but keep yourself positioned between the uprights. Alternate jumps with the bar and without it.

5. Continuing in the same training session, lay the uprights down and have your dog jump you again.

6. Remove the jump entirely. If your dog seems confused, hold the bar across your back as a visual cue.

7. Once your dog is comfortable jumping over your body, move away from him and stand with your back to him, arms extended. Look back at him and call "hup!" As your dog runs toward you, wait until the last second to crouch down. Very impressive!

VERBAL CUE
Hup
HAND SIGNAL

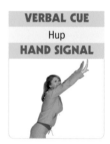

WHAT TO EXPECT: Athletic dogs can be jumping over you within a few weeks. Be sure your dog has good traction and is jumping with control. Send him to a **target** (page 145) after each jump to keep his trajectory straight. A few repetitions of this trick per day are enough to keep up your dog's skills without overdoing the stress on his body.

PREREQUISITES
Jump over a bar (page 108)

TROUBLESHOOTING

MY DOG IS LAUNCHING OFF MY BACK
Some dogs prefer to jump on your back on their way over while over while other dogs will do anything to avoid touching your back. Work in collaboration with your dog to develop the method that works best for the both of you.

BUILD ON IT! Build on this skill to learn **summersault/handstand vault** (page 114)!

TIP! Have a training goal for each session.

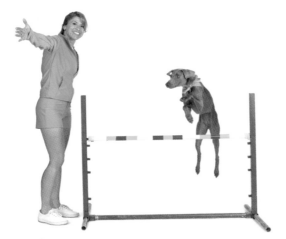

1 Send your dog over a 24" (61 cm) bar jump.

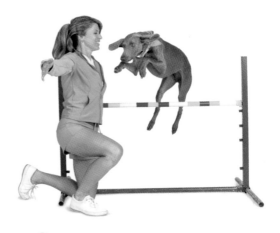

2 Crouch next to the upright as your dog jumps.

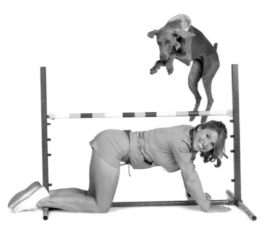

3 Kneel under the bar. Have a friend encourage your dog over if he seems reluctant.

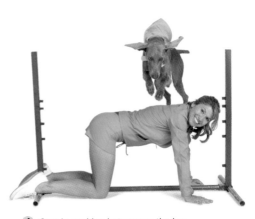

4 Stay in position but remove the bar.

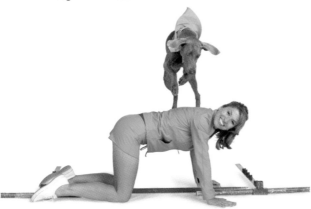

5 Lay the uprights down.

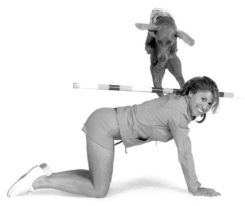

6 Remove the jump but hold the bar across your back as a visual cue.

Jump into My Arms

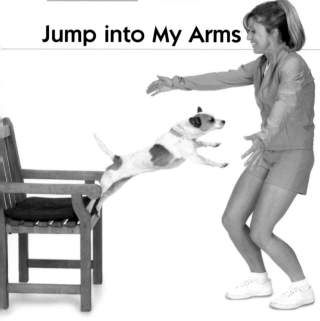

TEACH IT:

Your dog jumps toward your chest as you catch him in mid-air.

FORWARD JUMP (SMALL DOGS):

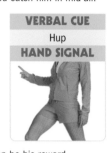

VERBAL CUE
Hup
HAND SIGNAL

1 Sit in a chair and encourage your dog to jump into your lap by patting your thighs and saying "hup!" A toy or treat should help motivate him. Be sure to catch him securely and praise and reward him while in your lap. If your dog enjoys being held, this can be his reward.

2 Gradually straighten up out of the chair. Press your back against a wall so your dog is confident in your stability as he uses your thighs as a push-off platform.

3 As your dog gains confidence, move away from the wall. Continue to bend your knees slightly to provide a ramp for your dog's jump. Be sure to catch him securely every time.

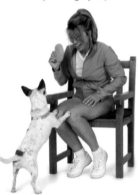 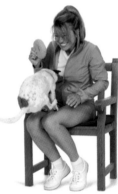

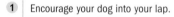
1 Encourage your dog into your lap. Praise him while there.

PREREQUISITES
Jump over my knee (page 109)

TROUBLESHOOTING

I DROPPED MY DOG!
Your dog is putting a lot of trust in you and needs to feel confident you will catch him securely. Go back to the basics and take care to catch him securely every time.

MY DOG DOESN'T HAVE ENOUGH ENERGY
If your dog is toy motivated, this will often inspire more enthusiasm than food. Tease him with a toy, and when he jumps, toss the toy a few inches and catch him!

TIP! You get enthusiasm by giving enthusiasm.

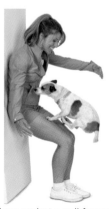 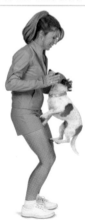

2 Lean against a wall for support. **3** Bend your knees slightly.

SIDEWAYS JUMP (SMALL OR LARGE DOGS):

1 Have your dog **jump over your knee** (page 109). Your dog should be on your left with your right knee raised. Hold your right hand high and away as a target for your dog, and use a toy if that helps.

2 Rise up slightly so your back knee is off the ground.

3 Continue to rise until you are in a position that causes your dog to jump high enough to be caught. When your dog is at the apex of his jump, lightly touch him with both hands in the position that will later become your catching grasp. Do not attempt a full catch the first time, as it will startle your dog. Increase the pressure and duration of your grasp, concentrating on carrying him through the path of his arc and releasing him to the ground.

4 Finally, catch your dog at the highest point of his jump, continuing to swing in the direction of his travel so as not to jolt him. Be sure his weight is distributed and excessive pressure is not caused on his neck or belly.

WHAT TO EXPECT: This trick requires a good amount of physical energy from your dog, as well as confidence in your ability to support him. Some dog/owner combinations may never be able to work this trick out.

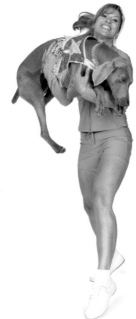

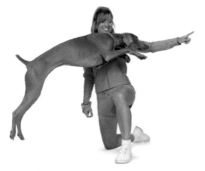

1 Have your dog jump over your knee.

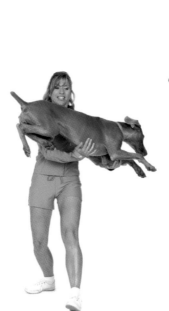

3 Lightly touch him as he jumps.

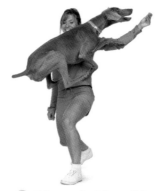

2 Raise your back knee off the ground.

4 Catch your dog at the apex of his jump.

Summersault/Handstand Vault

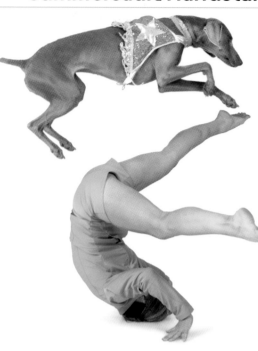

TEACH IT:

This spectacular trick requires precise synchronization and complete trust as you execute a summersault or a handstand while your dog vaults between your legs.

SUMMERSAULT:

VERBAL CUE
Summersault

1. Your dog already knows how to **jump over your back** (page 110) from behind you.
   Work with him now to jump the opposite direction. Face your dog and crouch down, arms extended, head bowed but tilted so you can make eye contact.

2. Add a slow-motion summersault. Walk toward your dog, arms raised straight up in the position that will later serve as your hand signal. Crouch down and tell your dog "summersault, hup!" After he jumps you put your hands on the ground, shoulder width apart, set your head between your hands with your chin tucked toward your chest, and roll forward. Practice this step several weeks before moving forward, as a collision with your dog could set him back significantly.

3. Your dog is now going to be asked to jump you while you are in mid-roll. He will need to calculate speed and distance and may not be successful at first. Remove your shoes in case of a collision. Keep your summersault slow but continuous. If your dog bails from the jump, try it again and praise him profusely when he is successful.

4. Finally, split your legs into a V for your dog to jump through! Your dog may at first be caught off guard when your legs separate, and collide with them. Teach him this configuration by starting your summersault in a straddle and keeping your legs split all the way through.

PREREQUISITES
Jump over my back (page 110)

BUILD ON IT! Have your dog carry a **baton** (page 116) while jumping!

TIP! Wear protective gear when performing the handstand.

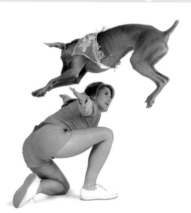

1. Face your dog as he jumps your body.

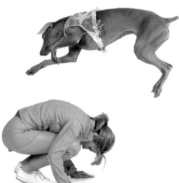

2. Finish a summersault after your dog has jumped you.

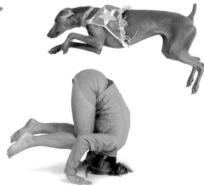

3. Try rolling while your is dog jumping.

HANDSTAND:

1 Practice a solo handstand; start in a lunge, hands extended up and slightly forward. Push with your front leg as your hands go to the ground and your back leg conversely goes up. Your feet should meet pointing toward the sky, then separate them into a wide V for your dog to jump through. Lower your head to the ground, tuck your chin toward your chest, and roll forward to finish.

2 Remove your shoes! Starting with a summersault vault, work incrementally to create a higher and higher summersault. Your first handstands should have your head lowering to the ground before your feet ever get straight up.

WHAT TO EXPECT: There will be few dog/trainer pairs that can pull this trick off. There are issues of size, jumping ability, confidence, and trust. If this is one you can master, you'll have the flashiest trick in town!

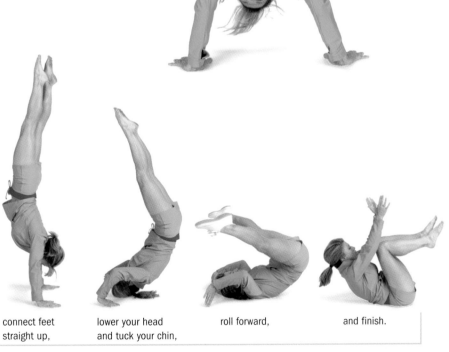

1 To perform a handstand, start in a lunge,   connect feet straight up,   lower your head and tuck your chin,   roll forward,   and finish.

Baton Jumping

PREREQUISITES
Jump over a bar (page 108)
Take it (page 25)

TIP! Your dog's safety comes first. Take a moment to survey the area, inspect your props, check for injuries, and consider anything that could go wrong.

TEACH IT:

Your dog jumps over your baton while holding one of his own. Creative positions can turn this trick into a real circus act!

1. Warm up with your dog **jumping over a bar** (page 108). Stand alongside the jump and use a sweeping motion with the arm farthest from your dog to signal him over.

VERBAL CUE
Hup
Baton

2. Remove the jump and hold just the bar parallel to the ground using the arm closest to your dog. Cue him to "hup" and lure him over with a treat in your other hand. If your dog tries to go around the bar, hold the other end against a wall.

3. Experiment with changing your body positions after every jump in a sequence of jumps. Decorate your bar or use a flashy baton.

4. Make a baton for your dog to hold. Select an object that your dog holds willingly in his mouth. A length of hose or irrigation tubing wrapped with colorful electrical tape works well, as does a tennis ball–textured throwing stick sold at pet stores. Associate the word "baton" with this object and have your dog **take it** (page 25) and hold his baton while he jumps!

WHAT TO EXPECT: Your dog can learn the basics of baton jumping in a few weeks. However, every new body position will require a learning period as you and your dog figure out the logistics. This collaborative effort is a true bonding experience.

"Sometimes, I don't want to hold my baton so I spit it out. Sometimes, I hold the very end from the corner of my mouth."

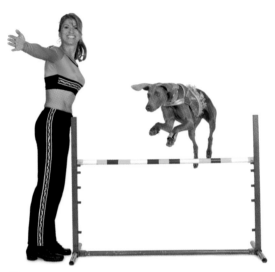

1 Use a sweeping motion to send your dog over the bar.

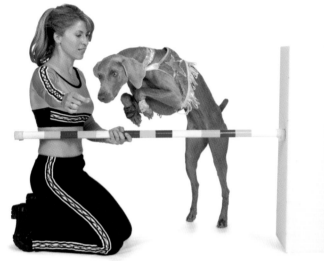

2 Hold the bar against a wall and lure your dog over.

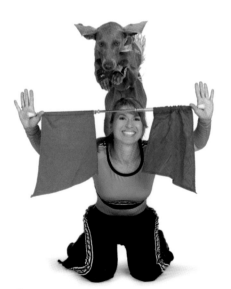

3 Use a flashy baton and experiment with different body positions.

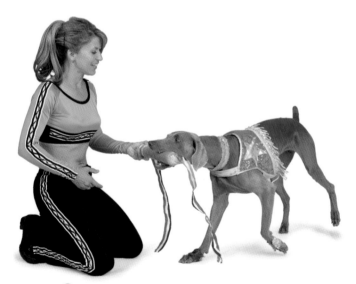

4 Make an easy-to-hold baton for your dog.

Jump Rope

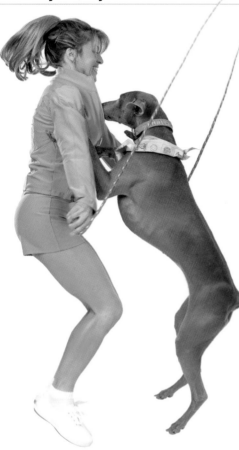

TEACH IT:

In the same way that you **jump rope**, your dog hops the rope as it is swung. Have two people hold the ends of the rope, or hold them both yourself as you jump with your dog.

1 Position your dog on a doormat or piece of carpet. Practice **jump for joy** (page 175) with your dog landing on the mat. Gradually work farther away from your dog, so you are able to stand several feet away while he continues to jump on the mat.

VERBAL CUE
Hup

2 Using a 7' (2 m), loose, lightweight rope, affix one end to an object at waist height. With your dog on the mat, slowly swing the rope back and forth to accustom your dog to it.

3 Cue your dog to **jump for joy** and attempt to swing the rope beneath him. Do not attempt a complete rotation with the rope. At first, reward your dog for jumping, whether or not the rope was successfully passed beneath him. Your dog will have to learn the rhythm of the rope. In the meantime, the timing of your cue will be essential to a successful jump.

4 Once your dog is able to clear the rope, it's time to add a second swing! If your dog has a long air time, or is shorter in body, you can swing the rope slower. Concentrate on swinging the rope low and sweeping it beneath him.

WHAT TO EXPECT: This trick can take the quickest learner months to achieve. Synchronization is key to your success, and it will take time for you and your dog to get on the same wavelength. Practice in short sessions, keep up the enthusiasm, and one day you'll find your dog is jumping rope! Once you've mastered a fixed-end rope jump, try holding both ends yourself, with your dog facing you.

PREREQUISITES
Jump for joy (page 175)

TROUBLESHOOTING

MY DOG JUMPS TOWARD ME AND OFF THE MAT
As he takes off to jump, make a move toward him, crowding him back. Reward him for landing on the mat.

MY DOG ISN'T JUMPING HIGH ENOUGH TO CLEAR THE ROPE
Try practicing with a hula hoop or stick. Your dog will feel it bump his ankles when he doesn't jump high enough.

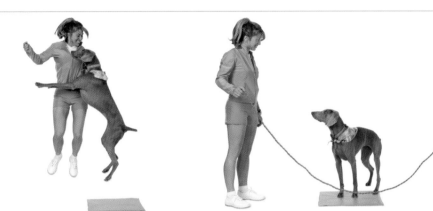

1 Practice **jump for joy** landing on a mat.

2 Familiarize your dog with the rope.

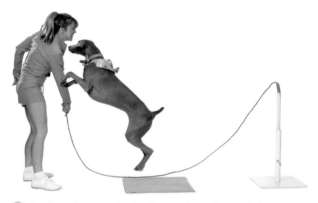

3 Cue **jump for joy** and swing the rope beneath your dog.

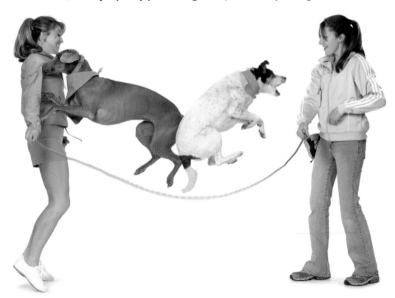

4 Add a second swing—or a second dog!

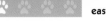

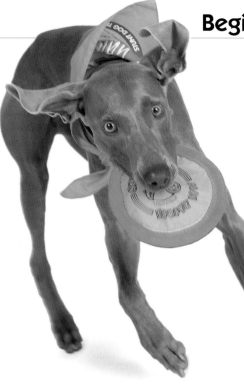

Beginning Disc Dog

TEACH IT:

Your dog's prey drive is engaged as he chases and catches a flying **disc**.

1 Use a flying disc specifically designed for a dog, such as a Hyperflite® or Frisbee® Fastback brand soft plastic disc, or a flexible Aerobie® Dogobie or Soft Bite Floppy Disc®. Hard plastic toy discs could injure your dog's mouth and teeth. Hold it parallel to the ground, fingers curled under the inside edge, with your index finger slightly extended. With shoulders perpendicular to your target, pull the disc across your body, take a step toward your target, and bring your arm across your body. Snap your elbow and wrist just before you release the disc.

VERBAL CUE
Frisbee or catch

2 Do not allow your dog free access to his disc—keep it hidden away to increase its desirability. When your dog is in a playful mood, spin the upside-down disc in circles. When he shows interest, throw a "roller"—rolling the disc along its edge like a wheel. End the play session while your dog's interest is still high.

3 Once your dog is chasing the disc, encourage him to bring it back to you by clapping your hands and calling to him to **come** (page 19). If he does not come, do not chase him but rather turn your back and ignore him.

4 Teach your dog to catch the disc in midair by throwing it in a low, flat trajectory. Do not throw it directly at your dog.

5 Your dog needs to **drop** (page 26) the disc after he returns to you. Try using two identical discs and throwing the second as soon as he drops the first.

WHAT TO EXPECT: Don't be discouraged if your dog does not immediately master an airborne catch, as it could take months to establish this coordination. Dogs under fourteen months should not be jumping for the disc, and all dogs should be checked by a veterinarian to ensure soundness. Dogs should jump in such a way that they land with four paws on the ground, rather than vertically, which can stress their spine and rear knees.

BUILD ON IT! Increase the difficulty by learning **disc vault off my leg** (page 122)!

TIP! 30 to 50 pound herding breeds are natural disc doggers!

"I like to chase my Frisbee. I jump up and chomp it. Gotcha!"

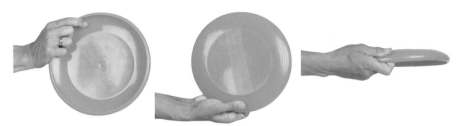

1 Good throwing form will send the disc in a low, flat, trajectory. Hold it parallel to the ground, fingers curled under the inside edge, with your index finger slightly extended.

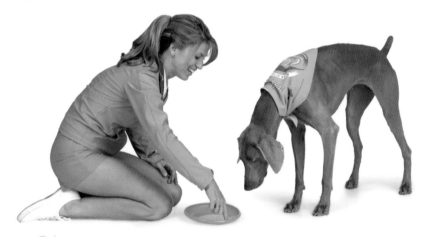

2 Spin the disc to attract your dog's interest.

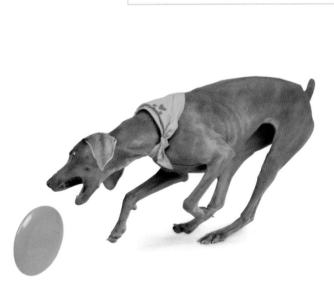

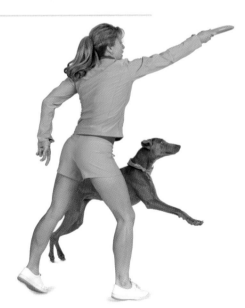

Roll the disc along its edge.

4 Teach your dog to catch a disc in midair.

Disc Vault off My Leg

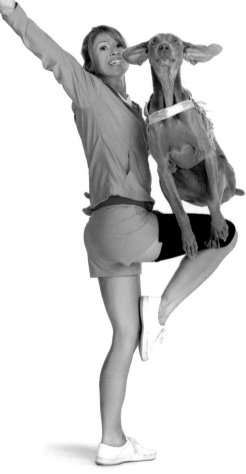

TEACH IT:

Your dog catapults off your raised thigh to catch a flying disc.

1 The first step is to combine two skills that your dog already knows: **jump over your knee** (page 109) and **catch a disc** (page 120). Assuming you are right handed, kneel with your dog on your left side and your right leg raised. Use your right hand to tap the disc on your thigh and then hold it high and to your right, encouraging your dog to use your thigh as a jumping platform to reach the disc.

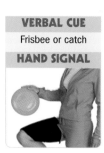

VERBAL CUE
Frisbee or catch

HAND SIGNAL

2 Once your dog is vaulting off your leg and taking the disc from your hand, start making small tosses. Remember to first tap your thigh with the disc to signal your dog.

3 Stand flamingo style, with your heel against your lower thigh. Start with your dog taking the disc from your hand and work up to small tosses. Now he's really getting air!

WHAT TO EXPECT: This trick requires accurate timing and placement of the disc, and it will be a learning process for both you and your dog. Keep your dog's motivation high by quitting with him still wanting more!

PREREQUISITES
Beginning disc dog (page 120)
Jump over my knee (page 109)

BUILD ON IT! Once you've mastered **leg vault**, try a chest vault or back vault!

TIP! A thigh wrap from a sporting goods store will protect you from scratches.

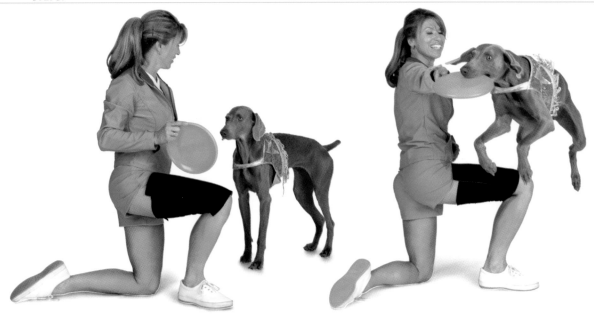

1 | With your dog on your left, raise your right knee. Have him lunge off your knee, grabbing the disc.

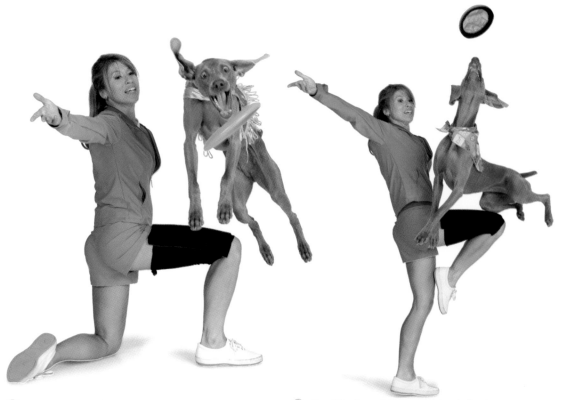

2 Start making small tosses.

3 Stand flamingo style for a greater challenge.

Chapter 8

Jumping through Hoops

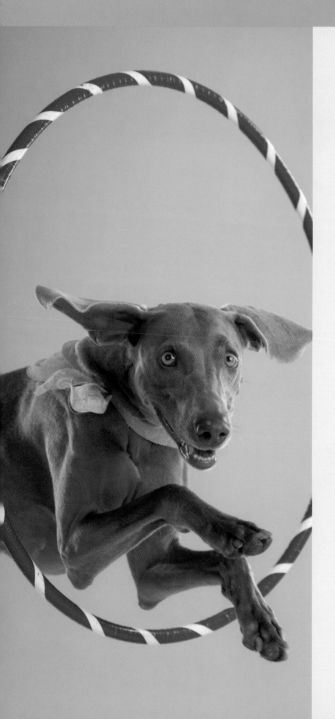

Flaming hoops
of death (actually hula hoops adorned with orange ribbon) are no match for your courageous canine, as he leaps and flies with confidence through spinning and rolling and paper-covered hoops!

The great thing about hoops is that any dog can learn tricks that use them and, with a little imagination, there is no end to the variety of tricks that can be composed with them: rolling hoops, circled arms for hoops, hoops lying on the ground, hoops over your back, under hoops, over hoops, little hoops, big hoops, and even two hoops!

Once learned, your dog will remember this skill forever. Dogs easily make the connection between other circular objects, such as the tire obstacle in the sport of agility and even your circled arms. Wherever you are, you can improvise a circle and delight your friends!

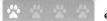 *easy*

Hoop Jump

TEACH IT:

Your dog jumps through a hoop, either fixed in place or handheld.

1 Remove the noisy beads within a toy hula hoop to make it less frightening for your dog. Hold the hoop on the ground with the hand closest to your dog, tell him "hup," and lure him through with a treat in your other hand. Praise him when he is through the hoop and allow him to have the treat. Some dogs are frightened to go through the hoop for the first time, in which case you can lead him through with a leash. To prevent your dog from going around the hoop, try placing it in a doorway.

VERBAL CUE
Hup

2 As your dog gets the idea, begin to raise the hoop off the floor. Dogs sometimes get tangled in the hoop, so be prepared to release it if you feel resistance.

3 Assuming your dog has the physical ability, raise the hoop again so that your dog must jump to get through it. Try giving him a running start or use your hand on the opposite side of the hoop to lure him upward. To reduce the risk of injury associated with your dog turning in midair, make a habit of tossing the treat in front of your dog rather than having him return to you for it.

WHAT TO EXPECT: Dogs usually get the hang of hoop jumping within a few weeks and do it enthusiastically. Decorate your hoop and use creative positions to enhance your performance.

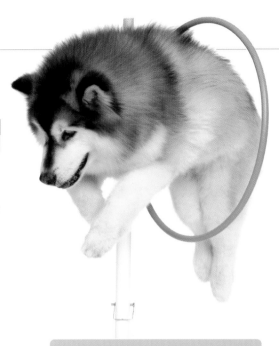

TROUBLESHOOTING

THE HOOP FELL ON MY DOG AND NOW HE IS FRIGHTENED OF IT!
Dogs pick up on your energy. Don't coddle your dog, just proceed with the lesson.

TIP! End your session on a happy note— ask you dog for a trick he already knows, and reward him for his brilliance!

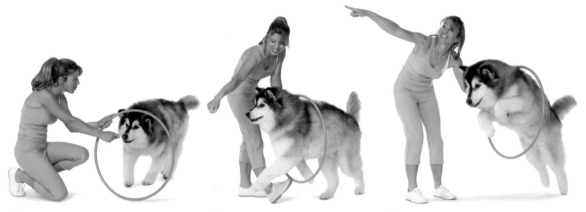

1 Lure your dog through with a treat.　　**2** Raise the hoop off the floor.　　**3** Toss the treat as your dog jumps.

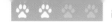

Jump through My Arms

PREREQUISITE
Hoop jump (page 125)

TROUBLESHOOTING

MY DOG IS TOO BIG TO FIT THROUGH MY ARMS
Widen your arms to allow space between your hands, or hold a flying disc or rope between your hands.

MY DOG JUMPS THROUGH THE HOOP, BUT IS RELUCTANT TO JUMP THROUGH MY ARMS
Some dogs are apprehensive about jumping close to your arms and head. Try alternating between the hoop and arm circles.

BUILD ON IT! Once he's mastered **jump through my arms**, it's only a short leap for your dog to learn **hoop jump over my back** (page 132)!

TIP! If your dog accidentally hurts you, don't let on! He'll be reluctant to perform a trick he fears might injure you.

TEACH IT:

Your dog jumps through a large circle formed by your arms.

1. Warm up with a few **hoop jumps** (page 125).

2. Gradually widen your arms around the hoop as your dog continues his jumps. Be careful to keep your head out of the way.

3. Continuing in the same session, set aside the hoop and cue your dog to jump through your arms only. A larger dog may require your hands to be disconnected. If your dog resists, go back to using the hoop.

4. Be creative; your dog can learn to jump through circles made with your arms or legs.

VERBAL CUE
Hup
HAND SIGNAL

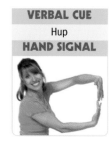

WHAT TO EXPECT: Dogs often take two steps forward and one step back with this trick. They may jump through your arms on the first day, but may require you to pick up the hoop the next day for a refresher.

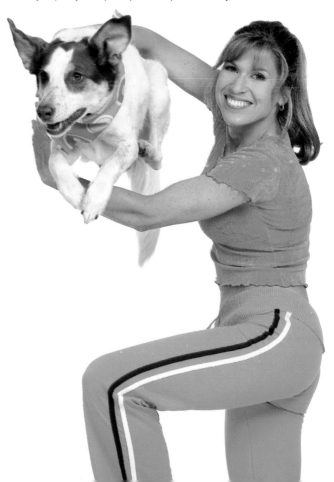

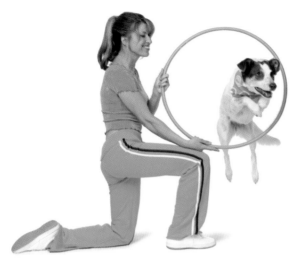

1 Warm up with hoop jumps.

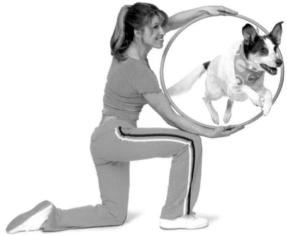

2 Widen your arms around the hoop.

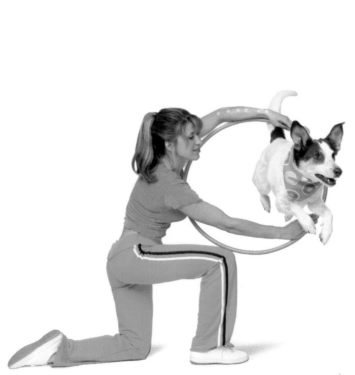

Keep your head out of the way as you widen your arms further.

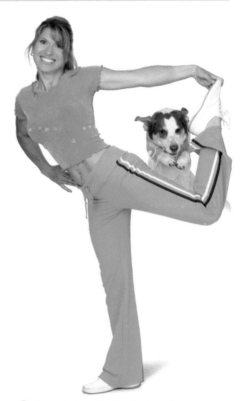

4 Form circles with other body parts.

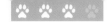

Double Hoop Sequence

TROUBLESHOOTING

MY DOG KNOCKS THE HOOPS EACH TIME, INSTEAD OF JUMPING CLEANLY
Your dog is cheating the jump. Take a step away from him right before he jumps, to encourage a powerful take-off.

TIP! Your dog always starts at your left, which means his hoop circle will be clockwise.

"Sometimes, I perform at the circus and wear a sparkly cape. There's lots of peanuts at the circus. I like peanuts."

TEACH IT:

Your dog runs circles around you jumping hoops in each of your arms.

HOOP CIRCLE:

VERBAL CUE
Hup

1. With your dog facing you, hold treats in your left hand behind your back, and a hoop in your right hand to your side. Tell your dog to "hup" and reward him with a treat from your left hand behind your back.

2. Pass the hoop to your left side and tell your dog to "hup" again, this time rewarding him in front of you from your right hand (a treat bag at your waist is convenient).

3. Introduce a second hoop. Without a free hand to guide your dog, the turn of your head will signal the correct hoop. Lean your left hoop on the front of your legs, and hold your right hoop to your side. Look toward the right hoop and move it slightly to emphasize it over the other hoop. Instruct your dog to jump through, and when he does, say "good" but do not offer a treat. Instead, immediately lower your right hoop to lean on the front of your legs and hold out the left hoop, turning your head in that direction and coaching your dog to go through. When he goes through your left hoop, give him a treat (it's OK to drop the hoops at this point).

4. When you are ready to try three jumps in succession, help your dog with his third jump by holding your right hoop angled in toward him after his second jump. Remember, your head turn will help guide him to the correct hoop. Always end the sequence with your dog passing through the left hoop, as you have eye contact in this position and will have fewer surprises.

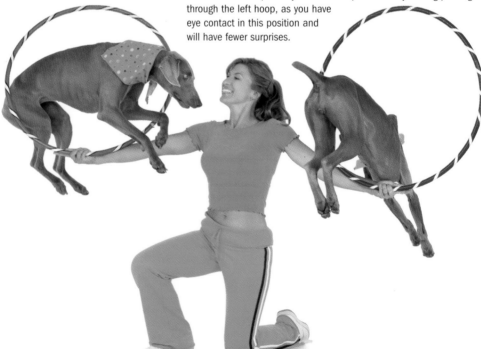

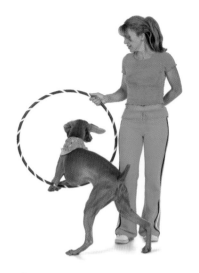

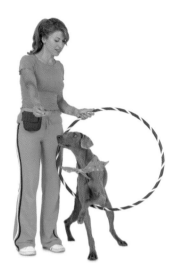

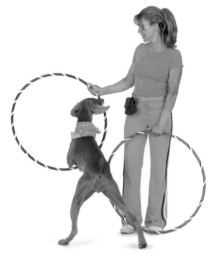

1 Hold the hoop at your right and give a treat behind your back.

2 Pass the hoop to your left side and reward in front.

3 Lean the left hoop against your legs.

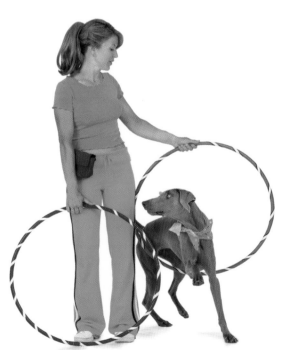

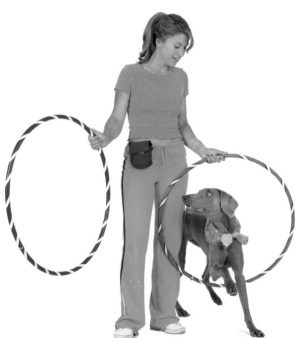

Lean the right hoop against your legs.

4 Angle your right hoop for the third jump.

(continued)

Double Hoop Sequence (continued)

PREREQUISITES
Hoop jump (page 125)
Helpful: Leg weave (page 170)

TROUBLESHOOTING

MY DOG DOES TURNS CLOCKWISE AFTER BOTH THE LEFT AND THE RIGHT HOOP

Your dog should turn to his left after jumping the right hoop, and vice versa. In this case, speed up your motion at the tail end of your dog's right hoop jump. Over time, he will learn to make a left turn in order to catch your next hoop.

TIP! Beware. Automobile antifreeze is lethal to dogs, even in amounts as small as a few licks. Dogs are often attracted to its sweet taste.

TEACH IT:

Your dog crossing back-and-forth jumping hoops as you walk.

HOOP WEAVE:

1 This trick will look a lot like a **leg weave** (page 170). Start your dog on your left side as you use your right hand to hold a hoop against the front of your right thigh. Step with your right leg as you tell your dog to "hup!"

VERBAL CUE
Hup

2 Immediately transfer the hoop to your left hand and hold it against your left thigh as you take a step. If your dog has trouble jumping in this direction, use your right hand to hold the hoop (still against your left thigh) and lure your dog through with a treat in your left hand. Practice until your dog can do a sequence of back-and-forth jumps as you walk forward.

3 It's time to introduce a second hoop. With your dog on your left, have your left hoop pressed against the front of your body so that your dog is seeing only its edge. Extend your right hoop forward on your right leg and have your dog jump through. As soon as he is through, reverse hoop positions to have your right hoop pressed against the front of your body as you take a step with your left foot.

4 Finally, keep both hoops parallel as you extend first one and then the other hoop while walking. Keep the nonactive hoop centered against its closest leg, so that your dog cannot jump through it.

WHAT TO EXPECT: As you train these tricks you will likely realize how debilitating it is to not have a free hand with which to signal. Eye contact is a powerful communication tool—use it! Dogs with a good hoop jump can pick up this variation in a matter of weeks.

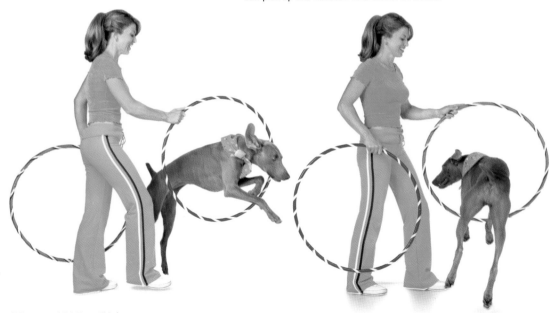

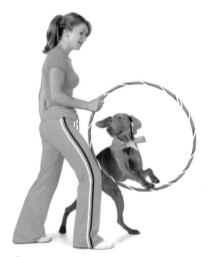

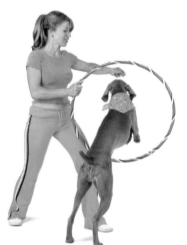

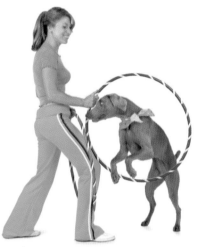

1 Hold the hoop with your right hand against your right thigh.

2 Step with your left leg. Lure your dog through with your left hand.

3 Hold the nonactive hoop flat against the front of your body.

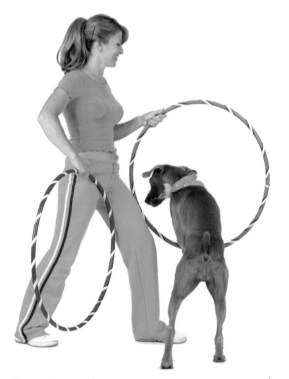

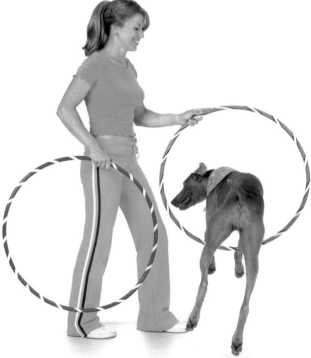

Reverse hoop positions.

4 Hoops are parallel. The nonactive one is centered against your leg.

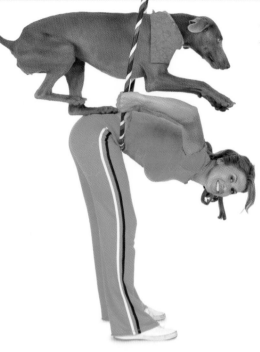

Hoop Jump over My Back

TEACH IT:

This trick combines a hoop jump with your dog jumping over your back.

1. Use a large hoop for this trick, so your dog has enough room to get through. Warm up with a few **hoop jumps** (page 125).

VERBAL CUE

Hup

2. Kneel down next to the hoop, with the arm closest to your dog encircling the bottom portion of the hoop. Gradually encroach into the circle with your head and shoulder.

3. Kneel on the ground with your head down and the hoop touching your stomach and pointing straight up. Turn your head so you can still see your dog.

4. Gradually rise up, with one foot on the ground and your hands holding the hoop about shoulder width apart. Keep your head down and the hoop pointing toward the sky.

5. In its final form, you'll be bent over with straight legs and the hoop pointing upward. To get into this position, put the hoop over your head and hold it parallel to the ground, touching your stomach. Position your feet apart for stability. Widen your hands on the hoop and bend over as if looking at your shoes.

WHAT TO EXPECT: This trick never fails to get "oohs" and "aahs!" When using a small hoop, your dog may step on your back.

PREREQUISITES
Hoop jump (page 125)
Jump over my back (page 110)

TROUBLESHOOTING

I GOT KICKED IN THE HEAD!
Keep your head down. Turn you head sideways if you need to make eye contact with your dog.

MY DOG CAN'T JUMP THAT HIGH
Execute the trick as in step four, while on one knee.

MY DOG JUMPED ON MY BACK AND STAYED THERE!
What a wonderful trick! Teach that behavior while your dog is offering it, and come back to the full jump another time.

TIP! Encourage your dog to trust you—be honest, be fair, be consistent.

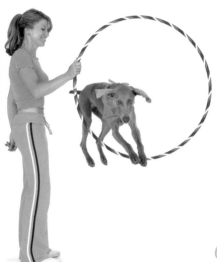

1 Have your dog jump through a large hoop.

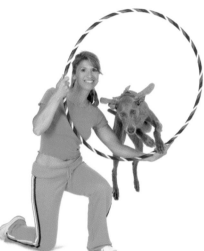

2 Encircle the hoop with the arm closest to your dog.

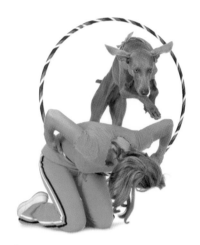

3 With the hoop touching your stomach, turn your head to look at your dog.

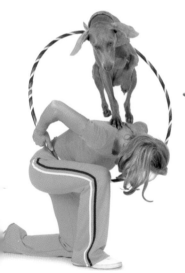

4 Rise to one foot and widen your arms on the hoop.

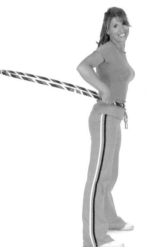

5 Get into position by placing the hoop against your stomach, feet apart...

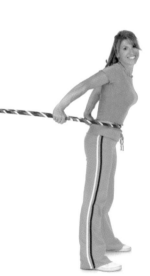

hands apart...

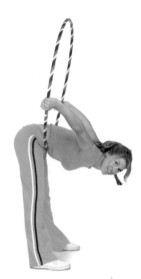

and bend over until the hoop is straight up.

Disobedient Dog—Under the Hoop

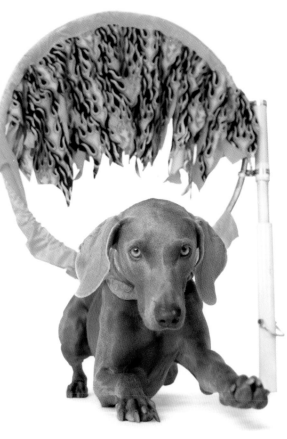

TEACH IT:

In this comedy routine, after an impressive introduction, you command your dog to jump through the flaming hoop! He instead crawls under it.

1. Set your hoop to a height higher than your dog normally jumps. He will be tempted to jump through it, but guide him carefully to instead walk under it.

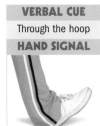

VERBAL CUE
Through the hoop
HAND SIGNAL

2. Set your dog on one side of the hoop while you stand on the other. Lift your toe and show him as you place a treat underneath. Instruct him to lie **down**, and then to **crawl** (page 144) under the hoop. Lift your shoe as he approaches to allow him to take the treat. You may have to keep repeating "down" and "crawl" throughout his travel.

3. Keep practicing as you gradually lower the height of the hoop and introduce the verbal cue.

4. In your performance, use a **target** object (page 145) to have your dog return to his original spot. Repeat this trick several times before telling your dog that the cute French poodle has just joined the audience, and subtly signaling him to jump the hoop's center. What a finale!

WHAT TO EXPECT: Your performance skill will be key to pulling this trick off. While your audience is distracted by your showmanship, your dog will take his cue from your lifted toe and your verbal cue "through the hoop," which he understands to mean "crawl under the hoop."

PREREQUISITES
Crawl (page 144)
Touch a Target (page 145)

TROUBLESHOOTING
MY DOG JUMPS THROUGH THE HOOP
Before giving your command, direct your dog's attention down toward the treat under your shoe.

BUILD ON IT! Continue this theme by teaching the **world's dumbest dog** trick (page 64).

"When I perform at the circus, I'm scared of the tigers. I know they're there because I can smell them."

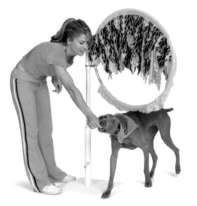

1 Lure your dog to walk under the hoop.

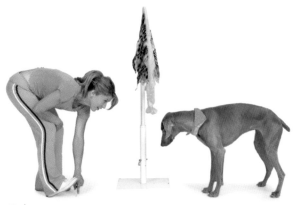

2 Show your dog as you place a treat under your foot.

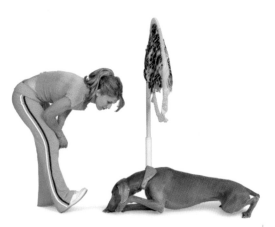

Instruct him to crawl until he is able to take the treat.

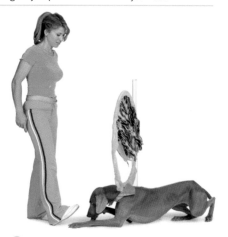

3 Lower the height of the hoop.

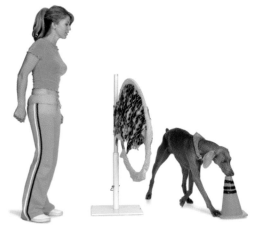

4 Have your dog return to his original spot by using a target object.

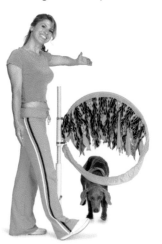

A little showmanship and your audience will be in stitches over your disobedient dog!

Rolling Hoop Dive

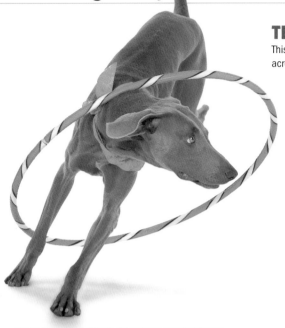

TEACH IT:

This flashy trick is also a great workout for your dog. As hoops are sped across the grass your dog chases them and dives through their centers!

1. Hold a large hoop in front of you and have your dog **hoop jump** (page 125).

> **VERBAL CUE**
> Get it!

2. Walk forward holding the hoop in front of you low to the ground, and accustom your dog to jumping through a moving object.

3. As you walk forward, send the hoop rolling in front of you a short distance and use an excited tone to tell your dog to "get it, hup!" Your dog may run to the hoop, and run back to you, not understanding. Keep alternating between walking with the hoop and sending it rolling. This is the hardest stage of learning, so keep up the enthusiasm!

4. This next step is training for you! Practice throwing a hoop fast and straight by balancing it on your collarbone as you grip the bottom underhanded. Concentrate on letting it roll out of your wrist.

5. Are you ready for the big time? Try multiple hoops. Assuming you are right handed, start with your dog on your left and throw your first hoop. Just before your dog runs through it, send the next hoop flying 90 degrees clockwise of the first. This will cause your dog to approach that hoop from the side, which will be easier for him. Keep throwing hoops in a clockwise direction until your dog has made a full circle! Way to shoot those hoops!

WHAT TO EXPECT: Dogs with a strong prey drive will love this trick. The chase is often reward enough that the dog does not need treats to be enthused. Quick-learning dogs will take several weeks before they are running through their first hoop.

"I close my eyes when I dive through the hoop."

PREREQUISITES
Jump through a hoop (page 125)

TROUBLESHOOTING

MY DOG KNOCKS THE HOOP OVER
A perpendicular angle of approach will help. Try the multiple hoop circle described in step five.

MY DOG IS SCARED
The secret is to engage his prey drive so that it outweighs his fear. His prey drive will increase with use.

BUILD ON IT! When your dog misses, teach him to go **through a hoop lying on the ground** (page 138).

TIP! Empty a water-filled hoop for a lightweight hoop that easily breaks apart at the seam if your dog gets tangled.

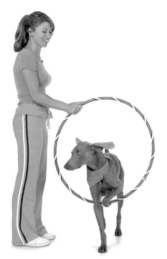

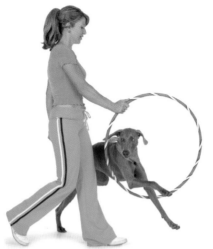

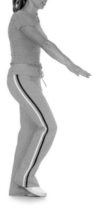

1 Have your dog jump in front of you.

2 Get your dog used to jumping through a moving hoop.

3 Roll the hoop a short distance as you walk.

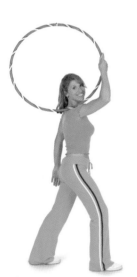

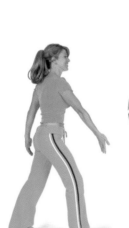

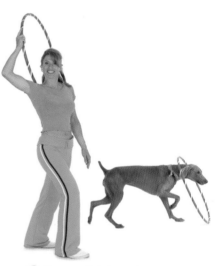

4 Balance the hoop on your collarbone. Hold it underhanded.

Roll the hoop down your arm and off your wrist.

5 Throw multiple hoops in a clockwise circle.

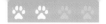
Through a Hoop Lying on the Ground

TROUBLESHOOTING

THE HOOP SLIDES AWAY FROM MY DOG
Grass works best when learning this skill, as other slippery surfaces may cause the hoop to slide.

MY DOG FETCHES THE HOOP INSTEAD OF GOING THROUGH
Your dog is eager and confused. Don't acknowledge the fetch, but keep prompting your dog to "go through."

TIP! Hoops come in different sizes, or make your own with irrigation tubing and connectors from the hardware store.

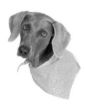

"Things that scare me: kitty in a bad mood, cotton balls. Nothing good ever happens with cotton balls."

TEACH IT:

Your dog maneuvers his way through a hoop lying on the ground. Dogs may invent different methods, any of which are acceptable.

1 Warm up with a few **hoop jumps** (page 125). Lower the hoop toward the floor, angling the top edge toward your dog so that he has to lower his head to walk through.

VERBAL CUE
Go through

2 Next, warp or kink your hoop so that it does not lie flat on the ground. Lift the leading edge to show your dog a familiar angle, and then lie it back down and instruct him to "go through." Hopefully, your dog will poke his nose under the kink and push his way under. You may have to reward your dog merely for poking his nose through, and work your way up to a full walk-through.

3 Over time, your dog will figure out which method works best for him; lifting the leading edge, the trailing edge, or even picking up the leading edge with his mouth and ducking under. The transition to a flat hoop shouldn't be too difficult.

WHAT TO EXPECT: This trick is easier to teach than you might expect, and it is impressive to watch! Practice every day and in a few weeks your dog should have the hang of it!

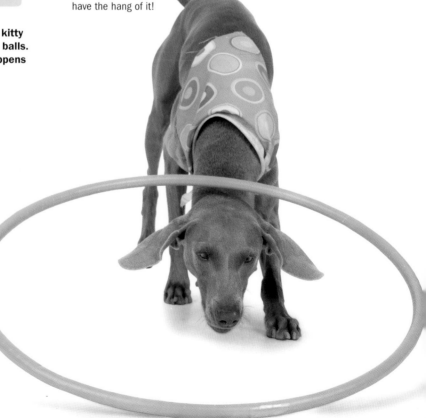

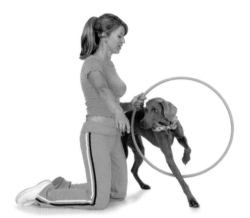

① Warm up with low hoop jumps.

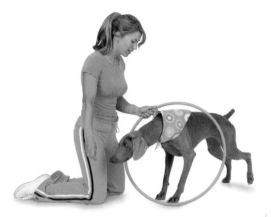

Set the hoop on the floor and angle it toward your dog.

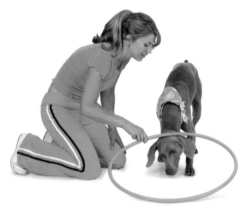

② Warp the hoop and lift it up slightly.

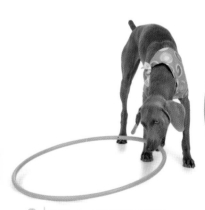

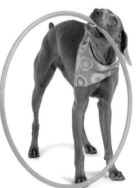

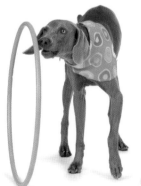

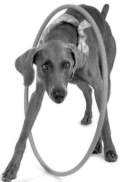

③ Dogs use different methods. Here, Chalcy lifts the leading edge,

balances the hoop upright,

ducks her head down,

and runs through!

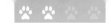
Paper-Covered Hoop

TROUBLESHOOTING

WILL NEWSPAPER WORK INSTEAD OF TISSUE PAPER?

Newspaper is significantly thicker than tissue paper, and dogs are more hesitant to jump through it. If you do use newspaper, cut a slit in the middle to give your dog a head start.

HOW DO I AFFIX THE PAPER TO THE EMBROIDERY HOOP?

Separate the two rings of the hoop, lay the paper across one ring, and press the other ring onto the first.

TIP! The goal of each training session is to get results a little better than the last time.

TEACH IT:

In this dramatic trick, your dog crashes through a paper-covered hoop.

1 A 24" (61 cm) embroidery hoop found at fabric shops offers a quick method of securing paper within a hoop. Practice a few **hoop jumps** (page 125) with it. Keep the hoop low to the ground, as it is smaller than a regular hoop and harder for your dog to clear.

VERBAL CUE
Hup or crash

2 Attach some tissue paper to the top edge of the hoop, putting a few rips in it so it doesn't look like a solid panel. Build your dog's confidence as he goes through.

3 Secure a sheet of tissue paper all the way across the hoop and tear a big hole in the middle. Use a treat to coax your dog through the hole. It may be easier to get him to walk through rather than jump. Praise him excitedly when he tears through the paper. Have him do a few more jumps through the hoop with the torn paper still hanging from it.

4 Attach a new piece of tissue paper to the hoop. This time, just make a small hole. Later, make just a slit.

5 Before you know it, your dog will be comfortable breaking through the paper on his own! Use two sheets of tissue paper side by side to get full coverage of the hoop and crumple the edges to keep it tidy.

"Sometimes, I just like to break things!"

WHAT TO EXPECT: This trick is a great confidence builder for dogs. They are often hesitant in the beginning, but within two weeks they are usually crashing through the paper like a bull in a china shop!

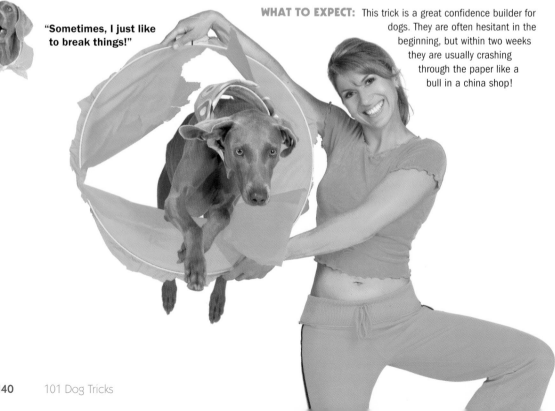

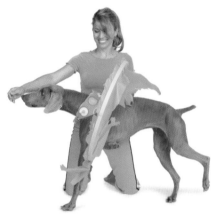

1 An embroidery hoop can be found at fabric shops.

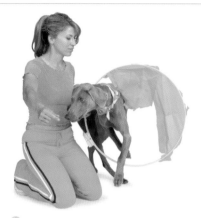

2 Attach tissue paper to the top edge and lure your dog through.

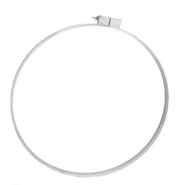

3 Cover the hoop with tissue paper, but make a big hole in the middle.

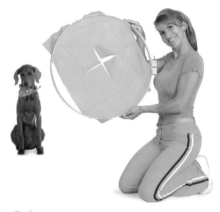

4 Graduate to a smaller hole,

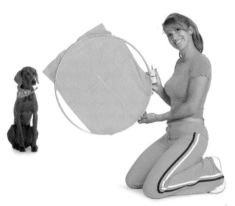

and then merely a slit in the paper.

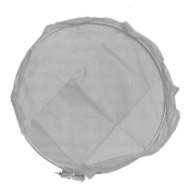

5 Use two sheets of paper and crumple the edges for a polished effect.

Chapter 9

Obstacle Course

Life is full of obstacles, and the sooner your dog learns to navigate them, the better! The obstacles in this chapter require logic skills and are often physically and mentally challenging. Some of them may even be scary for your dog at first, making his trust in you a necessary ingredient for success. Be patient and kind, encouraging but not forceful. Your dog may be hesitant at first, but once he comes through the other side of the tunnel (literally), he'll be a more confident dog!

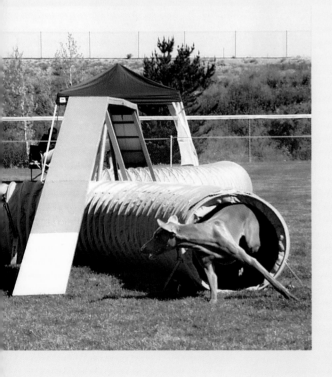

Dog's tend to dive into obstacles with wilder abandon than their humans. Make it your primary concern to look out for your dog's safety. Maintain regular veterinary checkups and inspect your dog's feet, ears, and coat often. Check your obstacles for nails, splinters, and places where your dog's foot could get stuck.

Work on a soft ground surface and be sure the obstacles have a high-traction surface. In jumping, your dog should land straight, not twisting, and largely horizontal. Increase difficulty gradually, as a bad experience may set progress back significantly. Combine several obstacles for a challenging run-through!

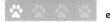
Tunnel

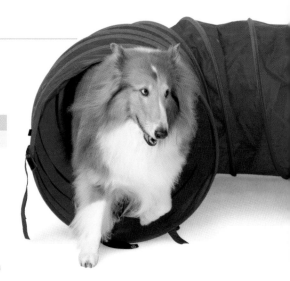

TEACH IT:

Your dog runs through a straight or curved **tunnel**. The tunnel is one of several obstacles in the sport of dog agility.

1 Allow your dog time to explore a short, straight tunnel in a familiar area. Set your dog at the opposite end and make eye contact with him through the tunnel. Coax him toward you. If he attempts to go around the tunnel, have a friend hold him and guide him in. Reward him with a treat at the tunnel exit.

VERBAL CUE
Tunnel

2 Once he is comfortable going through the tunnel, stand at the entrance with him, cue him with "tunnel," and guide him in. It often helps to get a running start. As he is running inside the tunnel, run along with him, encouraging him, so he can hear where you are. When he emerges at the other end keep running alongside him for a short way to encourage a speedy exit.

3 Put a bend in the tunnel. Your dog may try to make a U-turn inside and come back out the entrance, so keep your eye on him until you are sure he has committed.

WHAT TO EXPECT: Most dogs enjoy running through a tunnel and once accustomed to it, will do so every chance they get! Confident dogs can be running through the tunnel on their first day, while shy dogs may require more time.

TROUBLESHOOTING

CAN I PUT TREATS INSIDE THE TUNNEL?
Since the goal is for your dog to navigate the tunnel quickly, treats inside could create a bad habit of hesitating in the middle.

MY DOG IS SCARED TO GO INSIDE
Don't allow your dog's apparent fear to change your behavior. Be matter-of-fact about it and send him through. He will likely emerge a more confident dog!

TIP! You're so big! Get down at his level to engage your dog.

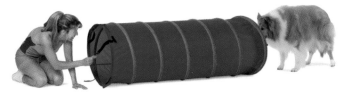

1 Coax your dog from the other end of the tunnel.

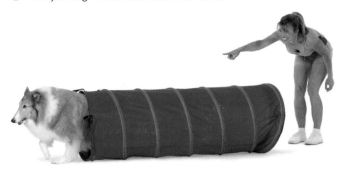

2 Send him from the entrance.

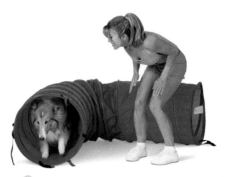

3 A running start propels your dog through a curved tunnel.

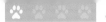

Crawl

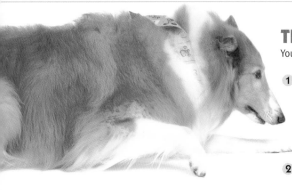

TEACH IT:

Your dog crawls forward, sliding his belly on the floor.

1. Your dog will be more willing to crawl on a comfortable surface such as grass or carpet. Put your dog in a **down** (page 16), facing you. Kneel on the ground and show your dog a treat hidden under your hand about 18" (46 cm) in front of him.

2. In a drawn-out voice tell him "crawl" as you slowly slide the treat away from him. He will hopefully take a crawl step or two with his front paws in an effort to follow the treat. Allow him to get the treat, while remaining down.

3. Once your dog is able to crawl following your treat, try standing several feet in front of him with the treat exposed under your foot. You may have to alternate saying "crawl" and "down" while he makes his way toward your foot. Your lifted toe will later become your dog's signal to crawl, keeping his attention low to the ground.

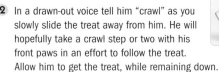

VERBAL CUE
Crawl
HAND SIGNAL

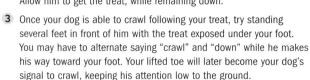

WHAT TO EXPECT: Many dogs are able to begin crawling in their first training session. Transitioning to using the verbal cue and foot signal, with no lure, often takes another few weeks.

PREREQUISITES
Down (page 16)

TROUBLESHOOTING

MY DOG STANDS UP
You are sliding the treat too fast.

MY DOG DOESN'T MOVE
He might believe he will be reprimanded for moving from his down. Keep your energy enthusiastic.

MY DOG HAS STARTED CRAWLING WHILE IN HIS DOWN-STAY!
Now that your dog knows this cue, tell him "no crawl" to stop this behavior.

BUILD ON IT! Use this skill to perform **disobedient dog** (page 134).

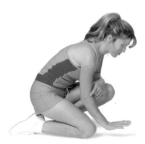

1. With your dog in a down, show him a treat under your hand.

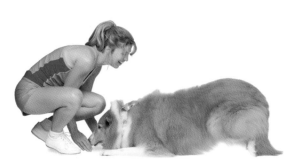

2. Slide the treat away from him as he crawls forward.

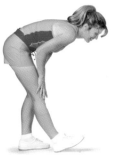

3. Place the treat under your foot to keep his attention downward.

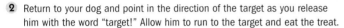

easy

Touch a Target

TEACH IT:

Your dog touches an object identified as a **target**. This useful skill has a variety of applications in trick training as well as dog sports and movie work.

1 In an empty environment, set up a **target** about 6' to 10' (1.8 to 3 m) away. The target can be a safety cone, plunger, or other unique object preferably one that your dog won't be tempted to take in his mouth. Show your dog as you or another person places a treat on the target. Get your dog's attention as you do this by saying "cookie" or whichever word he understands to mean a treat.

VERBAL CUE

Target

2 Return to your dog and point in the direction of the target as you release him with the word "target!" Allow him to run to the target and eat the treat.

3 After a few successful iterations, send your dog to the target without setting a treat on it. As soon as your dog touches the target, immediately praise him and give him a treat from your hand.

WHAT TO EXPECT: Practice ten iterations per day and within a week you may be able to send your dog to a target across the room!

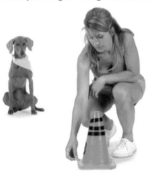

1 Place a treat on the target.

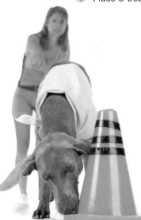

2 Reease your dog to get the treat.

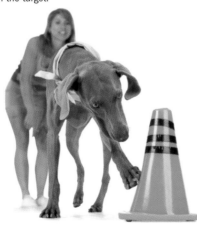

3 Send your dog to the target, and reward a touch.

TROUBLESHOOTING

IS MY DOG SUPPOSED TO TOUCH THE TARGET WITH HIS NOSE OR HIS PAW? While learning, either is acceptable. As you work with smaller and smaller target objects, your dog will find it easier to touch them with his paw, and will transition to this method on his own.

BUILD ON IT! Movie dogs use this skill to stop on a mark. Use a sheet of paper for the target. Gradually reduce the size of the paper, until a Post-it note is all that is needed.

TIP! Train your dog with a double command. "Target-sit" means to go to the target and sit.

"I teach a dog-tricks class at the park. I show the other dogs how to do stuff."

Obstacle Course   **145**

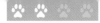
Under/Over

TEACH IT:

Your dog can be instructed to go either **under** or **over** any object.

1 Set up a bar jump or other obstacle at the height of your dog's back. Since he already knows how to **jump over a bar** (page 108), and is assuming that is what he is supposed to do, you'll want to begin this trick by training the **under** command. Set your dog on one side of the bar and lure him under by holding your treat low to the ground. Use the verbal cue often "under, good under!"

VERBAL CUE
Under
Over

2 Watch his body language and prevent him from jumping over the bar by blocking his path with your hand or by or holding his collar.

3 Lower the bar so that your dog has to duck down or crawl to get under. If your dog jumps over the bar, place him back in his original spot, taking care to lead him around the jump rather then letting him jump back over the bar a second time.

4 Now try with another object such as your outstretched leg.

5 Alternate the "under" and "over" commands to solidify the difference in your dog's mind.

WHAT TO EXPECT: This fun trick will keep your dog guessing as he awaits your instruction. In their eagerness, dogs don't always listen carefully and may require a month before they can concentrate enough to get this trick consistently right.

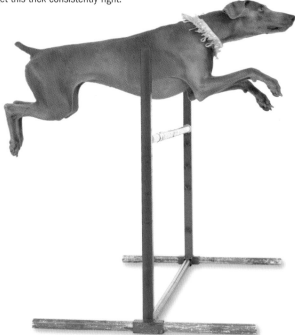

PREREQUISITES
Jump over a bar (page 108)

TROUBLESHOOTING

MY DOG COMPETES IN AGILITY. SHOULD I NOT TEACH THIS TRICK?
Dogs are smart and easily put behaviors into context. However, as an added precaution, you may want to teach this trick with an object other than a bar jump.

MY DOG KNOCKS THE BAR WHEN HE GOES UNDER
Some dogs use more finesse than others. Heavier objects such as tables and chairs should work well.

BUILD ON IT! It's time for a limbo contest! Once he's mastered **under**, see how low your dog can go!

TIP! Always do more **unders** than **overs** in a training session, as this will be the less instinctive one.

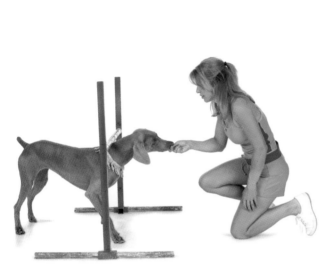

1 Set a bar at the height of your dog's back and lure him under.

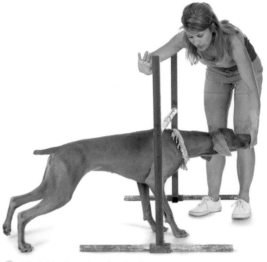

2 Block him from jumping the bar.

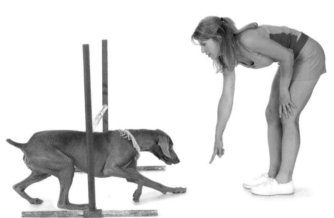

3 Lower the bar.

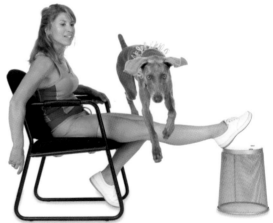

4 Try it with other objects such as your outstretched leg.

Teeter-Totter

"When my ears flip back, my owner says I have my party hat on."

TEACH IT:

The **teeter-totter** is an obstacle in the sport of dog agility that is weighted unevenly so that one end defaults to the down position. Your dog runs the length of the plank, balancing while it pivots midway.

1 With your dog watching, place several treats along the length of the plank.

<table><tr><td>**VERBAL CUE**</td></tr><tr><td>Teeter</td></tr></table>

2 Position a friend near the high end of the plank to keep it from making sudden movements. With fingers circling your dog's flat collar, start him at the low end and let him walk to the first treat.

3 As he continues to move forward, there will be a point at which his weight will pivot the plank. This is a good spot to place a treat, as it will slow him down. Your friend should guide the plank slowly and steadily as it pivots. Reassure him as you keep a firm grasp on his collar with his head forward. You don't want your dog to jump off the obstacle, so lift him off if he panics. Use lots of praise and encouragement with this new and unstable obstacle, and never use force as it will heighten an already present fear.

4 Once your dog gains confidence on the teeter-totter, your friend should allow the plank to move more freely, catching it only right before it hits the ground, so as to avoid a loud bang.

5 Let your dog try it on his own as you walk alongside him without touching him. Reward him while he is standing on the very end.

6 In the sport of dog agility, and for obvious safety reasons, dogs should not run so fast that they fly off the end of the plank before it touches the ground. Teach your dog to stop at the end by using a "wait" command or a **target** touch (page 145).

WHAT TO EXPECT: Most dogs are a little timid their first time on the teeter-totter, but they conquer their fear quickly with praise and treats! Don't force the issue—tomorrow is another day and your dog may feel differently about the obstacle then.

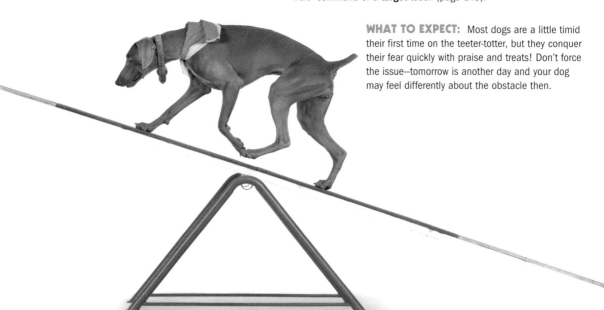

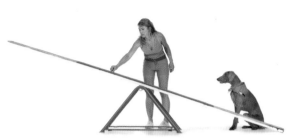

1 Place treats along the plank.

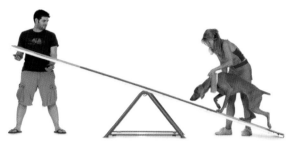

2 Guide your dog by his flat collar to the first treat.

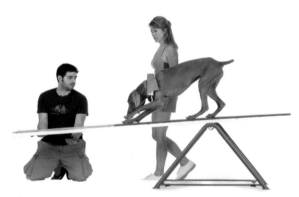

3 Keep control of your dog and the plank at the pivot point.

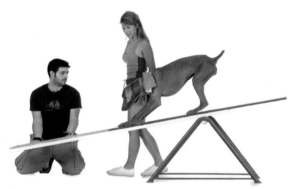

4 Catch the plank before it bangs down.

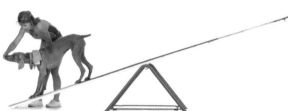

5 Walk alongside your dog as he goes it alone. Give a treat while he is standing at the end.

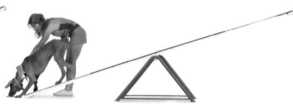

6 Teach your dog to touch a target at the bottom of the teeter-totter.

Weave Poles

MY DOG POPS OUT

Dogs that duck out of the poles are usually in too much of a hurry. Do not give him a reward, and start over from the beginning of the poles. Running right alongside him will help.

MY DOG MISSES THE FIRST POLE

Always stay behind the plane of the first pole when your dog enters, so as not to pull his attention away.

MY DOG MISSES THE LAST POLE!

The "last pole" syndrome happens when your dog responds to your body cues as you anticipate the end. Usually the cue is a slight lengthening of stride or a head turn as you locate the next obstacle. Visualize an endless line of poles and stay focused on them until after your dog has completed the poles.

BUILD ON IT! An off-side weave entry is where the handler is on the left side of the poles, while the dog still enters to the right.

TIP! Approach each training session with confidence. "Today, we're going to do it!"

TEACH IT:

Weave poles, an obstacle in the sport of dog agility, have your dog weaving in and out of a series of poles. The first pole is always passed along your dog's left shoulder, and the second along his right.

1 Start with only two poles (pointed plastic PVC poles can be stuck in the grass). With your dog on your left, give the verbal cue, lead him between the poles, and reward him.

VERBAL CUE
Weave

2 Stand parallel to the poles with your dog on your left and the poles to the left of him. Guide your dog to walk between the first two poles. Take a step forward, and reward him past the second pole.

3 Have your dog weave through a series of poles; lure him through with a treat, lead him through by his collar or short leash, or guide him through with your hand.

4 Begin with your dog a few feet behind and to the left of the first pole. Walk forward and guide him in and out of the poles by using your hand to "press" him away from you and "pull" him back.

WHAT TO EXPECT: Herding breeds tend to pick this skill up quickest and can be weaving on their own in several months. Other dogs often take six months to a year.

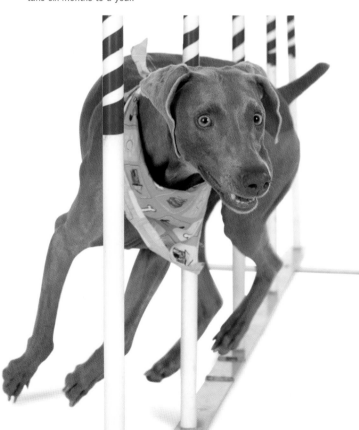

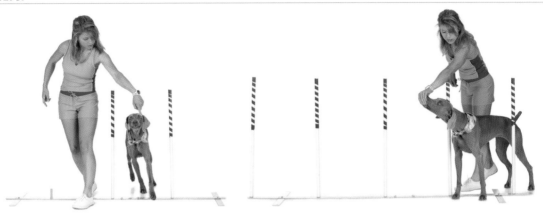

1. Guide your dog through two poles, angling so he passes the first with his left shoulder.

2. Start with your dog to the left of the poles. Reward him after the second pole.

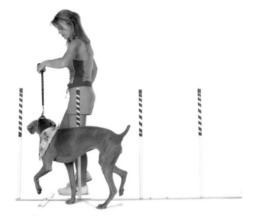

3. Guide your dog through a series of poles using a treat, a leash, or your hand.

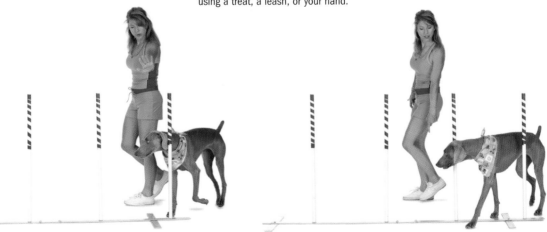

4. Walk alongside your dog as you use your hand to "press" and "pull" him through the poles.

Climb a Ladder

TEACH IT:

Your dog maneuvering his front and back paws up the steps of a ladder.

1. Cover the steps of a sturdy ladder with a nonslip surface. Using a treat, lure your dog to place his front paws on one of the lower rungs. Do not touch or confine your dog, as he will want to feel he has an escape route. Raise the treat to encourage him to place his front paws higher.

   VERBAL CUE
   Climb

2. Still luring your dog's head upward, use your other hand to coax his back paw onto the first step.

3. Your dog is now in a precarious position, so guard his body to help stabilize him. Continue to raise the treat higher and allow him to position his front paws himself. Practice only 5 minutes per session, and allow your dog to break between attempts.

4. Once your dog is comfortable climbing the steps, place your treat at the top of the ladder to motivate a speedy ascent!

WHAT TO EXPECT: Climbing a ladder requires not only coordination and strength but also confidence. Take it slowly as a misstep or frightening experience can set your dog back.

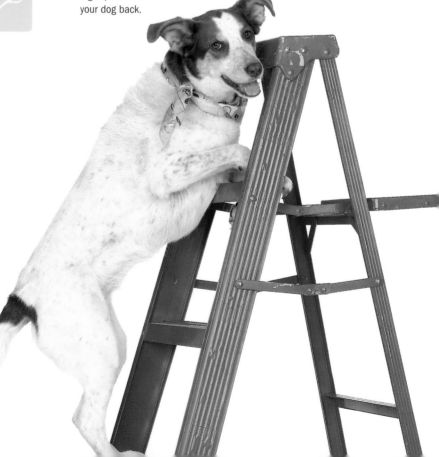

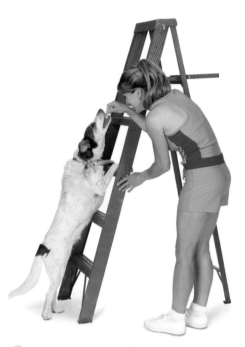

1 Lure your dog to place his front paws on a rung.

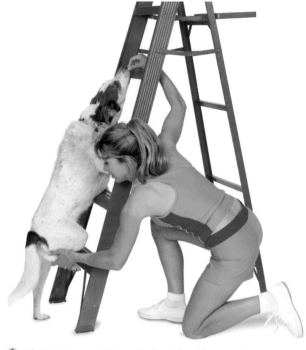

2 Lift his back paw while continuing to lure him upward.

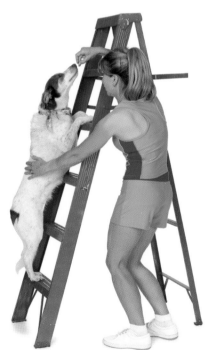

3 Guard his body while raising the treat.

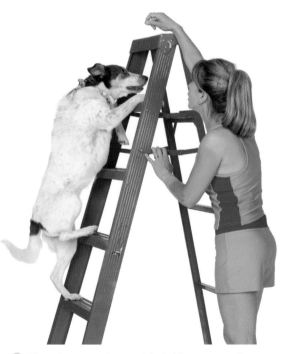

4 Place the treat at the top of the ladder as a reward.

Roll a Barrel

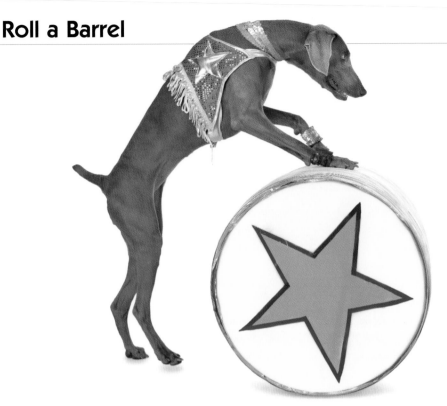

TIP! Increase your dog's motivation by varying the consistency, amount, and types of treats. Sometimes, offer a goldfish cracker, sometimes nothing, and sometimes a jackpot of treats!

TEACH IT:

There are several variations of **rolling on a barrel**, including the dog rolling it with his front paws, his rear paws, or all four paws. He can roll it forward or backward.

ROLLING WITH FRONT PAWS:

VERBAL CUE
Roll

1. With your dog at your side, steady the barrel and lure your dog upward with a treat. Reward him for placing his front paws on the barrel.

2. Do the same while standing on the opposite side of the barrel.

3. Now start rolling the barrel. A grass surface is preferable since it prohibits fast motion and provides a soft landing. Place your foot on the barrel with your leg outstretched. Once your dog's front paws are up on the barrel, lure his head forward with a treat. Roll the barrel toward you by pulling with your foot. Praise and reward your dog for shifting his paw backward.

4. As your dog improves, use your foot to roll the barrel sporadically. Roll it a bit, and lure him forward until he rolls it a bit himself. At this point, your dog will have to comprehend a difficult concept—walking his front paws backward while his back paws walk forward!

5. If your dog stops rolling the barrel, gently tap his paws with your foot to encourage him to move them back. Praise and reward.

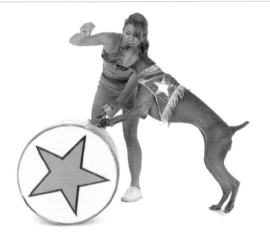

1 Lure his front paws up.

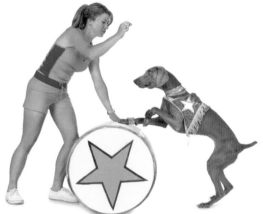

2 Now try the opposite side.

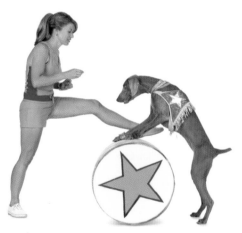

3 Roll the barrel toward you,

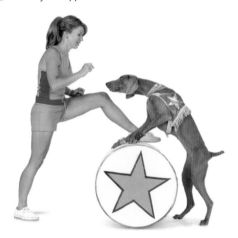

luring his head forward,

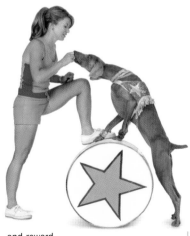

and reward.

(continued)

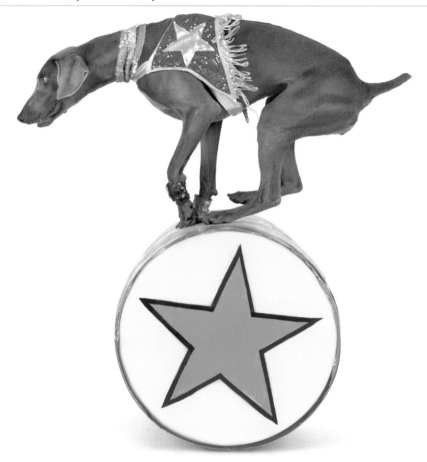

TROUBLESHOOTING

MY DOG JUMPS ON OR OVER THE BARREL
Use your body to block the other side of the barrel.

TIP! This exercise teaches body awareness, which is valuable for any dog.

ROLLING ON TOP:

1. With your dog on the opposite side of the barrel, hold it stationary with your foot and lure him on top. Be ready to steady him when he jumps. Allow him to nibble a treat from your hand, keeping your hand stable, as he will press against it for balance. Try to get him to stay on top of the barrel for as long as you can.

2. Roll the barrel 6" (15 cm) away you using your foot. Be prepared with your hand or body to block your dog from jumping off. When he takes a step forward, praise and reward.

3. Roll the barrel sporadically until your dog is doing it on his own!

WHAT TO EXPECT: This is not a trick your dog can learn in a weekend. It may take twenty sessions for him to roll the barrel with his front paws, and could take months for him to find his balance with all four paws on top. Certain breeds are better built for this trick—long-legged and top-heavy dogs will have the hardest time.

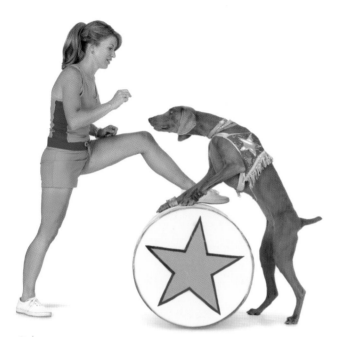

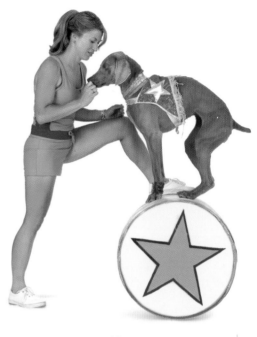

1 Hold the barrel with your foot and lure your dog up.

Let him nibble a treat while on top.

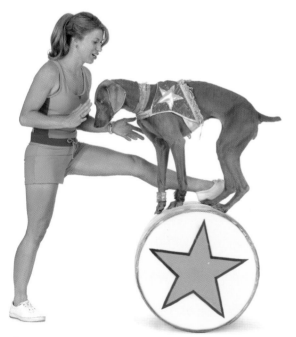

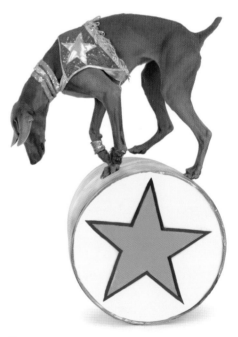

2 Roll the barrel away from you. Be prepared to block your dog from jumping off.

3 With practice your dog will be doing it on his own!

Chapter 10

That Dog Can Dance!

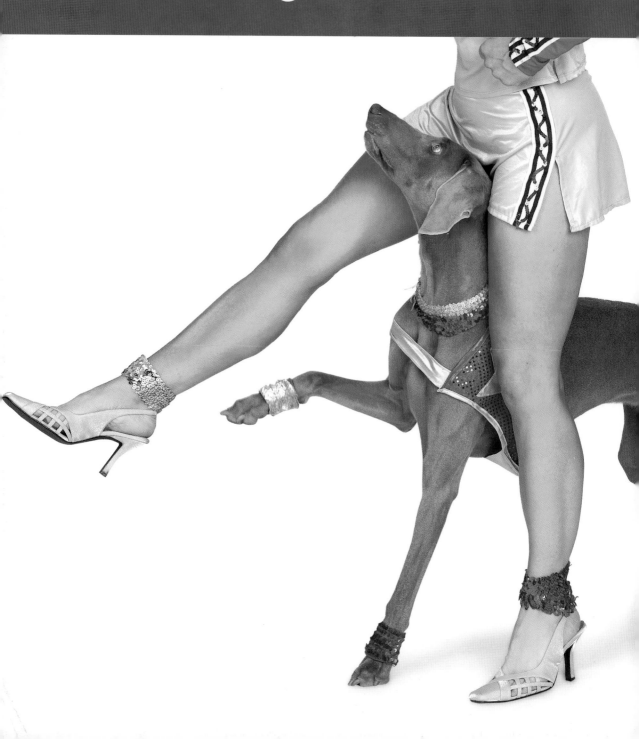

Active

people have active dogs. And if you notice your pooch has a paunch, it might be time time for some exercise … for the both of you!

The sport of canine freestyle has popularized the tricks in this chapter by chaining them together into dance sequences. Choreographed to music, you and your dog execute synchronized spins, leg kicks, and dance steps. This is a wonderful way to work as a team with your dog and develop the bond that comes from mutual reliance.

Eye contact is key to a synchronized performance. Hold bits of cheese in your mouth and spit them to your dog as a reward to encourage his attention.

Don't underestimate the importance of your performance! Little flourishes will transform a dull series of behaviors into a lively show!

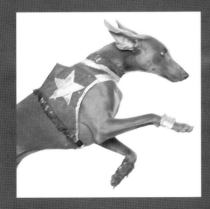

Heel Forward and Backward

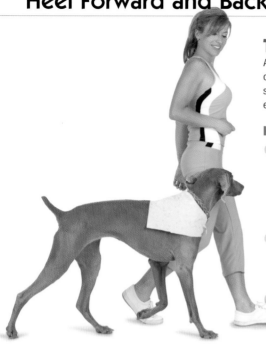

TEACH IT:

A dog at **heel** walks at the handler's left side. In the sport of dog obedience, the dog automatically sits when the handler stops. In the sport of freestyle (dog dancing) the heel is less rigid, focusing more on eye contact and gait.

HEEL:

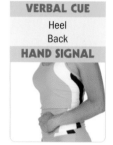

VERBAL CUE
Heel
Back
HAND SIGNAL

1. With your dog on a loose leash at your left side, say "heel" and walk forward, stepping first with your left foot. This step will later become your dog's signal to heel. Always give the verbal command first, before starting your motion.

2. Reward your dog periodically for a good effort, remembering to reward at the time when your dog is in the correct position—with his shoulder aligned to your left leg.

3. When preparing to stop, slow your gait, plant your left foot, and bring your right foot up to meet it. Pull up on the leash and say "**sit**" (page 15).

HEEL BACKWARD:

4. With your dog on a short leash at your left, tap his chest with your right foot while cueing "back." Reward him for taking a step back. As you reward him, don't cause him to step forward by offering the treat too far in front of him. Practice heeling backward alongside a wall to keep your dog straight.

WHAT TO EXPECT: In obedience classes, most dogs will be heeling nicely on leash by the end of eight weeks. Heeling is an art form, however, that can always be refined!

PREREQUISITES
Sit (page 15)

TROUBLESHOOTING

MY DOG LAGS BEHIND
Pat your leg and use peppy encouragement, or break into a jog.

MY DOG PULLS FORWARD
Give a quick jerk on the leash followed by release of tension. This should immediately bring your dog back into position, at which time you praise him with "good heel."

BUILD ON IT! Continue to practice **heeling** until your dog can do it off-leash!

TIP! The more your dog knows, the easier he will learn.

HEEL:

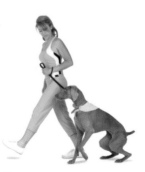

1. Command "heel" and step with your left foot.

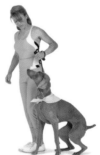

3. Command "sit" when you stop.

HEEL BACKWARD:

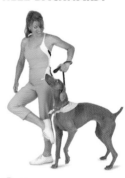

1. Use your right foot to tap your dog backward.

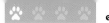 *easy*

Back Up

TEACH IT:

Your dog **backs up** in a straight line away from you.

1 Stand in a hallway facing your dog while holding a treat in your closed fist directly in front of his nose. Press gently on his nose while walking toward him giving the verbal cue "scoot." As your dog takes a few steps backward, praise and release the treat. If he squirms use your foot opposite the wall to guide that side, or place an ex-pen to create a narrow chute.

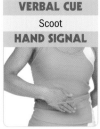

VERBAL CUE
Scoot
HAND SIGNAL

2 Once your dog is getting the hang of this, start to decrease dependence on the nose push by instead walking in toward your dog while raising your knees to gently bump his chest. Use your hand to signal him backward.

3 Over time, take smaller steps forward, while continuing to raise your knees to pressure your dog backward. Walk over to him to give a reward, or toss one to him, rather than calling him back to you.

WHAT TO EXPECT: In a week, your dog could be walking backward following your treat. In another few weeks, you may be able to stand stationary while he backs up.

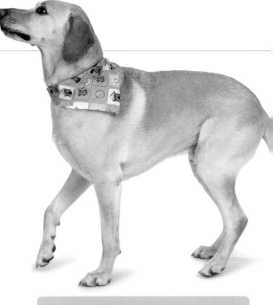

TROUBLESHOOTING

MY DOG BOWS
You may be holding the treat too low. Keep it no lower than nose height.

MY DOG SITS
Holding the treat too high will lift your dog's nose and cause him to sit. Bump him with your knee to cause him to hop backward.

TIP! Hand signals are more powerful than words. Be aware of your signals.

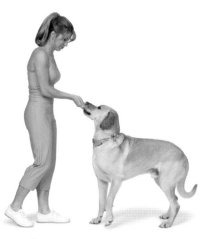

1 Press a treat against your dog's nose.

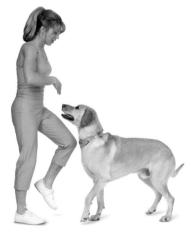

2 Raise your knees as you walk toward your dog.

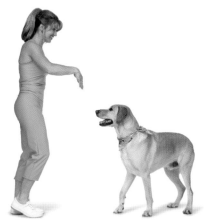

3 Take smaller steps forward while continuing to raise your knees.

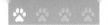
Spin Circles

BUILD ON IT! Teach military turns—while **heeling** (page 160), cue your dog "around" as you turn left 180 degrees. Continue heeling in the opposite direction.

"I love going to the pet store. I find things under the shelves!"

TEACH IT:

Your dog **spins** either a left or a right full circle.

SPIN:

1. Begin with your dog facing you, hiding a treat in your right hand. Move your hand to your right, in a large counter-clockwise circle, slowly luring your dog while telling him "spin." Release the treat at the end of the circle.

2. As your dog improves, diminish your hand signal until it is merely a flick of your wrist.

3. Add some pizzazz—a spin is doubly exciting when you mirror your dog's movement. As your dog spins, cross your right foot in front of your left and pivot on your toes until you've spun completely around. (And you thought your dog was going to do all the work!)

4. Reach around by using your left hand to trace a clockwise circle.

WHAT TO EXPECT: Practice ten times per day, and your dog should be following your hand easily within a week. In a month, he can be spinning on command!

VERBAL CUE
Spin (counter-clockwise)
Around (clockwise)

HAND SIGNAL

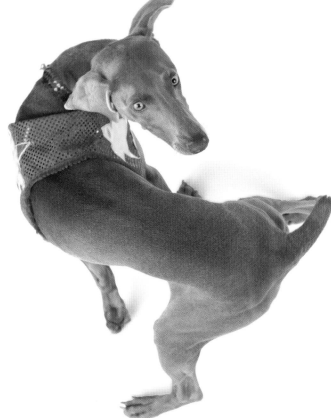

SPIN:

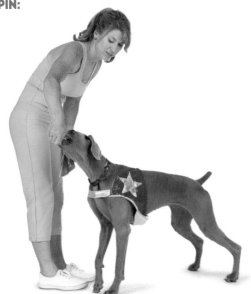

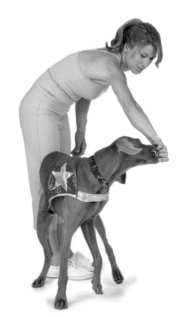

1 Hide a treat in your right hand.

Move your hand directly to your right, and trace a large circle.

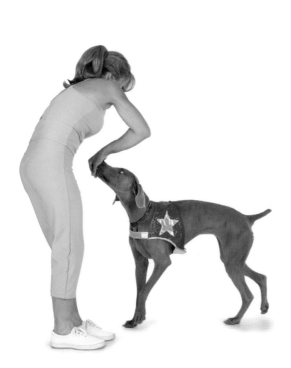

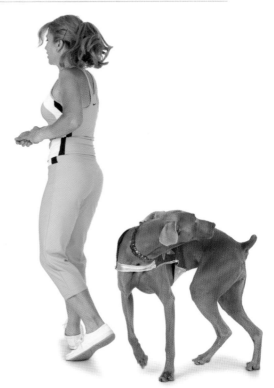

Release the treat when the circle is complete.

3 Spin with your dog for added pizzazz!

Take a Bow

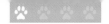

TROUBLESHOOTING

MY DOG SITS INSTEAD OF BOWING
You are holding the treat to high. Start at nose height and press toward your dog's hind paws.

MY DOG LIES DOWN
Release the treat sooner. You may have to reward before his elbows touch the ground. If this does not solve the problem, position your foot on the floor under his belly.

BUILD ON IT! Once you've mastered **take a bow**, use a similar action to learn **say your prayers** (page 42)!

TIP! Give your dog an ear massage, inside and out. Arf!

TEACH IT:

Your dog **bows** by keeping his back legs upright, while bowing down his front until his elbows touch the floor.

1 Have your dog stand facing you. Hold a treat in your fist at nose height.

2 Gently press your hand into your dog's nose and downward, while giving the verbal cue.

3 As soon as your dog's elbows touch the floor, release the treat and back your hand away.

VERBAL CUE
Bow or Curtsy
HAND SIGNAL

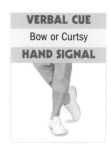

WHAT TO EXPECT: Practice this trick six to ten iterations per day. Remember to quit while it's still fun.) After one to two weeks your dog should be bowing easily when you press a treat to his nose. Gradually lighten your touch on his nose, and soon your dog will be bowing on his own. Thank you! Thank you very much!

"I do a curtsy, because I'm a girl dog."

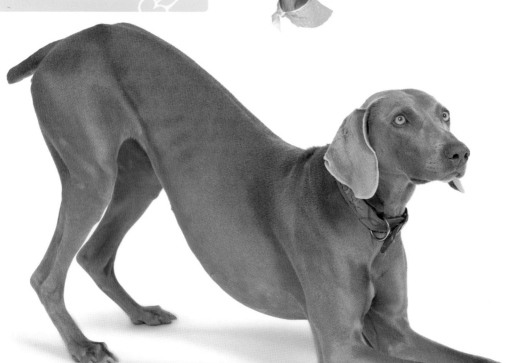

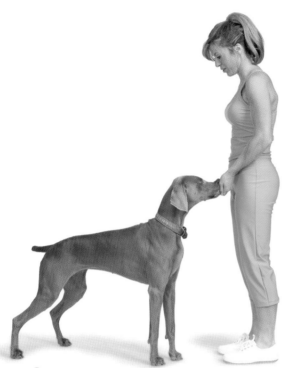

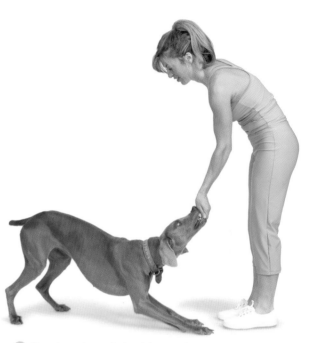

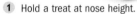

1 Hold a treat at nose height.

2 Press toward your dog and downward.

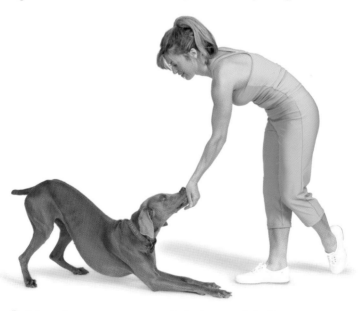

3 Release the treat as soon as your dog's elbows touch the floor.

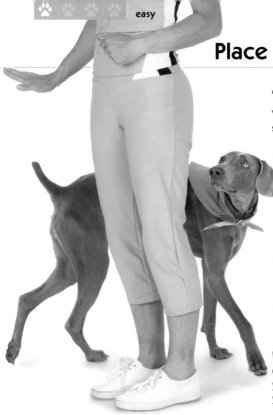

Place (circle to my left side)

TEACH IT:

Your dog circles behind you to end sitting at your left side. This can be the start to a heeling drill or the end to an obedience test.

1. Stand facing your dog with his leash in your right hand.

2. Say "place" and take a step back with your right foot, pulling your dog toward your right side and behind you. Keep your left foot planted throughout this exercise.

3. Transfer the leash to your left hand while returning your right foot next to your left and pulling your dog into position at your left side.

4. Pull up on the leash and tell your dog to **sit** (page 15). Praise and reward your dog in this position.

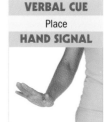

VERBAL CUE
Place
HAND SIGNAL

WHAT TO EXPECT: This trick is quite impressive as your dog shows off his obedience training. In its final stage, keep both feet planted while your off-leash dog responds to your cue to circle behind you and sit at your left side.

PREREQUISITES
Sit (page 15)

TROUBLESHOOTING

MY DOG IS SO SLOW!
As your dog is passing behind you, take an extra step or two forward and tell him to "get it up!"

I FEEL LIKE I'M JUST PULLING MY DOG AROUND ME
You are conditioning your dog to the movement. At first, you *are* pulling him around, but over time his muscle memory will take over.

TIP! It takes approximately 100 repetitions for a dog to learn a new trick. Have patience!

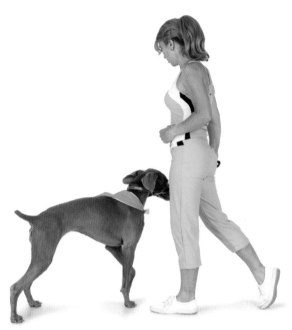

2 With the leash in your right hand, step back with your right foot.

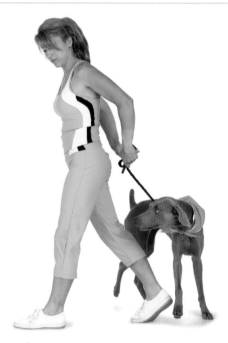

3 Transfer the leash to your left hand.

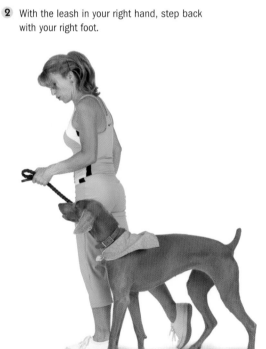

Return your right foot next to your left as you pull your dog into position at your side.

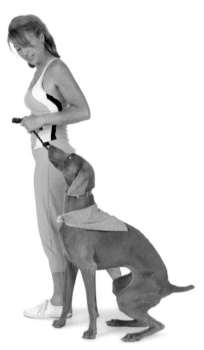

4 Pull up on the leash as you command your dog to sit.

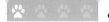
Side (swing to my left side)

TROUBLESHOOTING

MY DOG SITS TOO FAR IN FRONT OR BEHIND ME
You'll be surprised at how your body position can affect your dog's sit. Slight adjustments to your left shoulder position will bring your dog forward or back.

MY DOG SITS CROOKED
Tap his left haunch as he is sitting to bring it in tight.

TIP! Consistency is key to success. Practice motions solo before involving your dog.

TEACH IT:

Starting facing you, your dog makes a tight circle, almost pivoting on his front paws, to come to a sit at your left side.

1 Face your dog holding his leash in your left hand.

2 Tell him "side" and step back with your left foot, pulling your dog to your left and slightly away from your body. Your right foot remains planted throughout this exercise.

3 Circle your dog clockwise, bringing his head in the space where your left leg used to be.

4 Bring your left leg back into position and have your dog **sit** (page 15) at your side. Reward your dog while he his sitting.

WHAT TO EXPECT: With practice, your off-leash dog will jump into position while you stand in place. Energetic dogs may learn on their own to hop into position rather than circle.

VERBAL CUE
Side
HAND SIGNAL

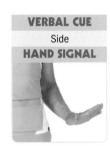

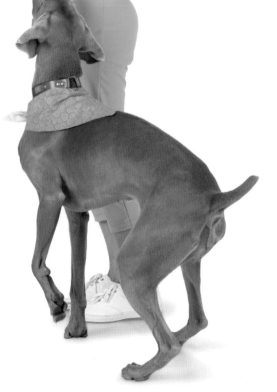

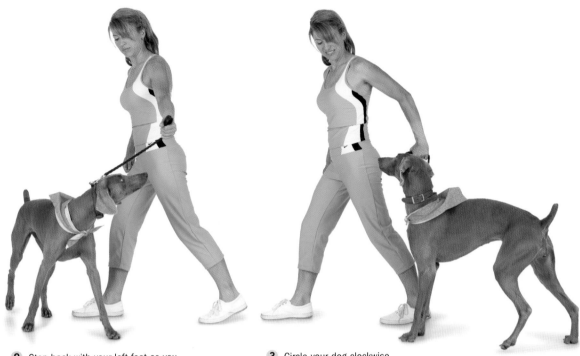

2 Step back with your left foot as you pull your dog back and away.

3 Circle your dog clockwise.

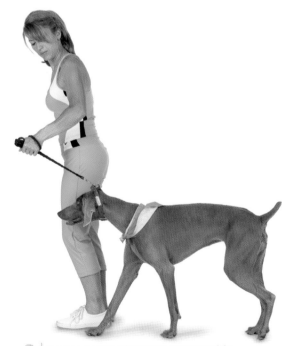

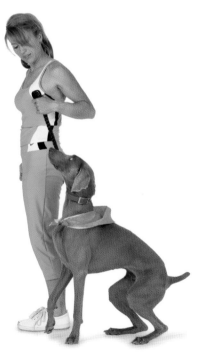

4 Bring your left leg forward to meet your right.

Have your dog sit.

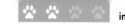

Leg Weave

TROUBLESHOOTING

MY DOG RESISTS WALKING BETWEEN MY LEGS

Start with the **peekaboo** trick (page 52) to reinforce this position.

I'M HAVING TROUBLE WITH MY COORDINATION

Instead of treats, use a tab leash to guide your dog. Step with your right foot and pull the leash between your legs with your right hand.

MY DOG IS TOO EXCITED AND NOT FOLLOWING MY HAND SMOOTHLY

This is not uncommon in the beginning. Focus on one weave at a time, and reward each.

MY DOG IS TOO TALL

Unless you're looking to take a tumble, this probably isn't a trick for a Great Dane!

BUILD ON IT! Once you've mastered **leg weave**, use a similar action to learn **figure 8's** (page 172)!

TIP! Always start **leg weave** by stepping with your right foot. Stepping with your left foot is a signal to heel.

"On weekends I have just so much to do!"

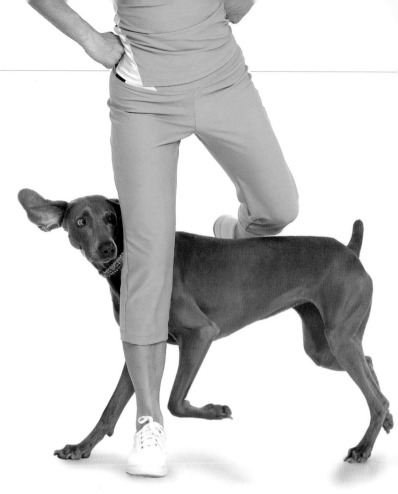

TEACH IT:

Your dog crosses back and forth between your legs as you walk. This trick is not for the uncoordinated!

1. Start with your dog sitting or standing at your left side. Hold several small treats in each hand.

2. Take a big step with your right foot and drop your right hand straight down between your legs while giving the verbal cue. As your dog crosses between your legs, reward him with a treat from your right hand.

3. Take a step with your left foot and drop your left hand straight down while giving the verbal cue. Again, treat your dog when he noses your left hand.

4. Repeat the steps.

VERBAL CUE
Weave
HAND SIGNAL

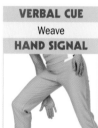

WHAT TO EXPECT: Practice this trick in five-minute sessions, once or twice per day. After two weeks, your dog should be following your hand smoothly, and you can require several successful weaves before treating. Keep practicing until your dog speeds through your legs with no hand guidance at all!

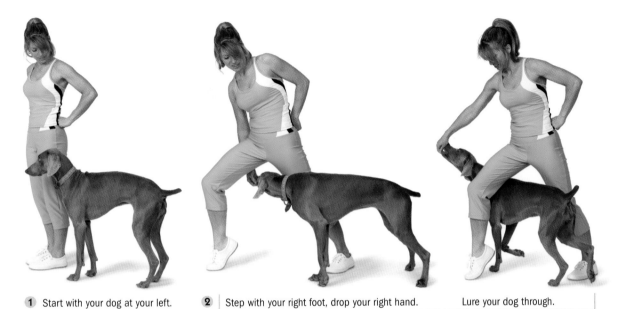

1 Start with your dog at your left.

2 Step with your right foot, drop your right hand.

Lure your dog through.

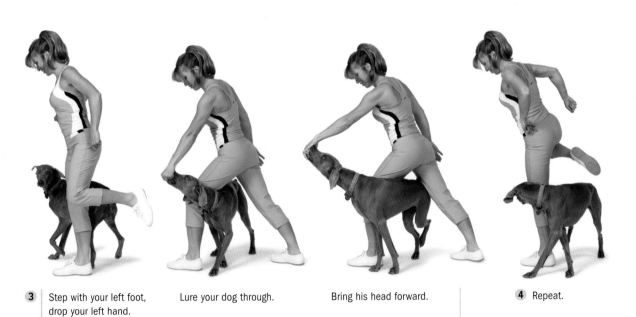

3 Step with your left foot, drop your left hand.

Lure your dog through.

Bring his head forward.

4 Repeat.

Figure 8's

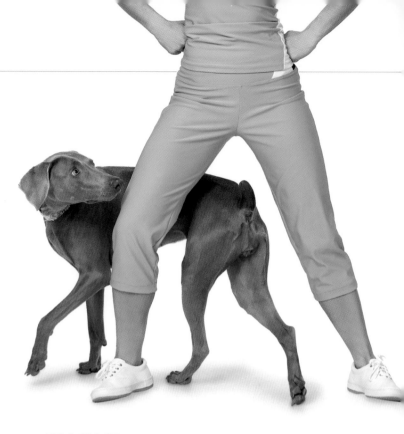

PREREQUISITES
Leg Weave (page 170)

TROUBLESHOOTING

WHICH WAY IS MY DOG GOING THROUGH MY LEGS?

Because this is adapted from the **leg weave**, your dog always starts at your left side and crosses through your legs, front to back, and then circles your right leg first. Your dog will always be passing through your legs front to back.

BUILD ON IT! For an impressive dance sequence, have your dog do several figure 8's, and after he passes through your legs in anticipation of circling your right leg, close your legs and use your right hand to cue him to **spin** (page 162).

TIP! Figure 8's are a good part of your stretching and warm-up routine to help prevent injury before exercise

"We have a kitty named JoJo. You have to watch out for her because she swats when you go around corners."

TEACH IT:

As you stand with your legs apart, your dog runs figure 8's through them.

1. Warm up with a **leg weave** (page 170).

2. Next, try the **leg weave** while taking steps that are wider apart but shorter going forward. Continue to use the "weave" cue.

3. Transition to taking steps in place, with your legs wide apart, without making forward progress. Continue to lift each foot to cue the dog, and say "weave." Use an imaginary leash to "pull," or guide, your dog through your legs from front to back.

4. Finally, keep your feet planted but lunge to each side as your dog crosses between your legs. As he crosses between your legs in preparation for circling your right leg, your right leg should be bent, and he should see your right hand guiding him through your legs and toward your right leg. Now is the time to change your verbal cue to "cross." Have him do several figure 8's in a row before treating. Give him the treat as he is doing the action, rather than after he has stopped.

VERBAL CUE
Cross
HAND SIGNAL

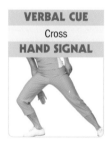

WHAT TO EXPECT: With a reliable **leg weave**, your dog can pick up the figure 8 in a few days. As you continue to train, you will be able to do it without lunging and with your hands on your hips.

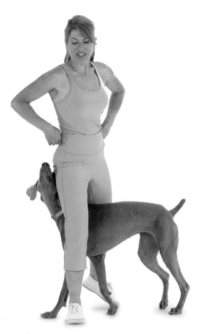 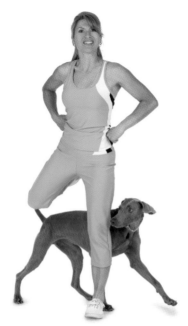 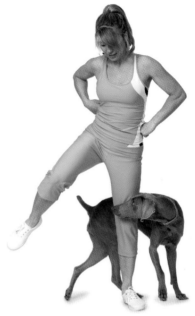

1 Practice a leg weave.

2 Make your steps shorter and wider apart.

3 Using a wide stance, alternate lifting each foot in place.

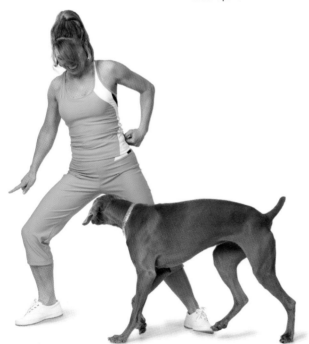 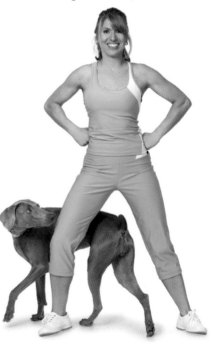

4 With feet planted, guide your dog through your legs, front to back.

Stand in place with hands on hips while your dog runs figure 8's around you!

Moonwalk

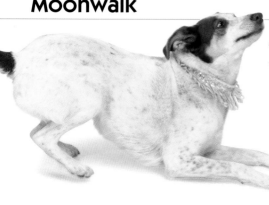

TEACH IT:

When **moonwalking**, your dog scoots backward while in a bow position.

1 Face your dog with him in a **down** position (page 16). In much the same way you taught him to **back up** (page 161), push your knee toward him while giving the "scoot" cue. He will likely try to stand up, so guard his shoulder blades with your hand to keep him down. Reward even a small scoot backward.

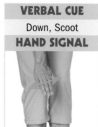

VERBAL CUE
Down, Scoot
HAND SIGNAL

2 Start to stand up straighter, and minimize your knee action. Continue to guard your dog's shoulders, pushing him down every time he rises.

3 Stand in place while giving the hand signal and verbal cue. If your dog rises to his feet, tell him "down" and then "scoot." You may have to alternate these cues repeatedly.

WHAT TO EXPECT: This adorable dance move can be learned in a few weeks by a dog with a solid **back up**. Dogs will often try to cheat by rising up, so be vigilant about form!

PREREQUISITES
Down (page 16)
Back up (page 161)

TROUBLESHOOTING

MY DOG DOESN'T MOVE BACKWARD
When first teaching **moonwalk**, don't use the word "down," but rather just prevent your dog from rising up by guarding his shoulders. Telling him "down" may confuse him into thinking he is not supposed to move.

TIP! When your dog needs medicine, a spoonful of peanut butter will help the pill go down.

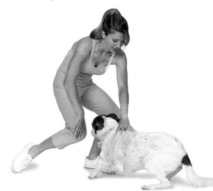

1 Guard his shoulder blades while pressing your knee toward him.

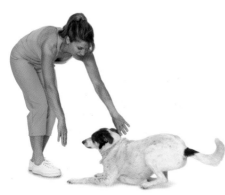

2 Minimize your knee action, while continuing to guard his shoulders.

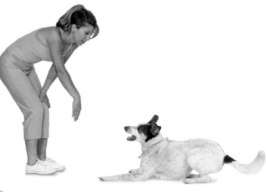

3 Stand in place while giving the cue.

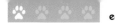
Jump for Joy

TEACH IT:

When **jumping for joy**, your dog jumps straight up, landing in the same spot. You are going to need all your enthusiasm for this one, because no one jumps for joy alone!

1 While your dog is in a playful mood, hold a toy or food high in the air and tease him with it. Encourage him by jumping along with him! Reward even small jumps at first.

2 Once your dog has the hang of jumping along with you, tone down your jumping motion by merely crouching down and standing up while using the verbal cue and hand signal.

3 Eventually, your dog will be able to jump for joy on cue, but your enthusiasm will be key.

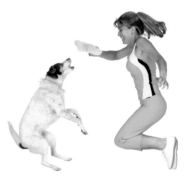

VERBAL CUE
Jump
HAND SIGNAL

WHAT TO EXPECT: Some dogs are naturally bouncier than others—terriers, Australian shepherds, and whippets, to name a few. Other dogs may need much more encouragement to put forth the effort.

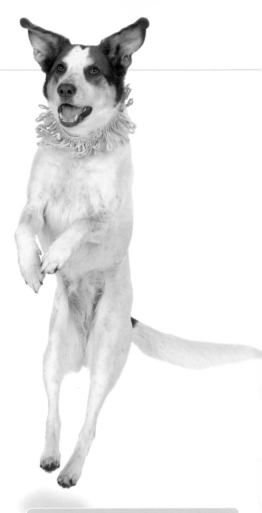

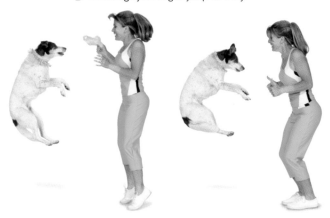

1 Encourage your dog to jump for a toy.

2 Tone down your jumping motion.

3 Your dog will jump on cue.

TROUBLESHOOTING

MY DOG IS LAZY AND WON'T JUMP
Your job as a trainer is to instruct and MOTIVATE! Get those springs in your legs and bounce right along with your buddy. Use your most excited "happy voice" to get him amped.

BUILD ON IT! This skill is the first step in learning to **jump rope** (page 118)!

TIP! Practice on grass or other surface that provides traction. The ideal jump should be straight and smooth.

Chorus Line Kicks

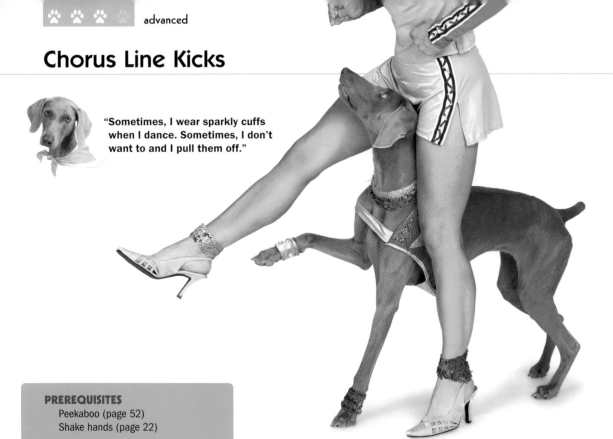

"Sometimes, I wear sparkly cuffs when I dance. Sometimes, I don't want to and I pull them off."

PREREQUISITES
Peekaboo (page 52)
Shake hands (page 22)

TROUBLESHOOTING

MY DOG WALKS FORWARD, COMING OUT OF HIS PEEKABOO
Your dog wants to see your face. Lean over so he can see you. Use your hand to block his chest if he moves forward, and remind him to "peekaboo."

MY DOG JUST STANDS THERE, NOT MOVING HIS PAWS
Sometimes, it takes a few iterations to get your dog in the swing. Try a few times, "shake, paw, shake, paw" while leaning to the side each time, which will slightly push your dog's weight to one side, encouraging him lift his opposite paw.

TIP! Play a favorite song on the stereo and dance with your dog!

TEACH IT:

When performing **chorus line kicks**, your dog stands between your legs and high kicks his front paws in sync with your kicks.

① Starting in a **peekaboo** position (page 52), reach your left hand down and a little forward and tell your dog to "**shake**" (page 22). Do not hold a treat in your hand while you do this, as it will guide his nose rather than his paw. Reward him instead with a treat from your treat bag at your waist. Repeat with "**paw**" while signalling with your right hand.

② Add your corresponding leg kicks to enhance the effect. Your hand signals will eventually become subtle flicks of two fingers by your hip, which will be your dog's cue (rather than your kicks).

③ Try variations of this trick with your dog facing you or at your side.

VERBAL CUE
Shake, paw

HAND SIGNAL

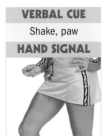

WHAT TO EXPECT: This jazzy trick can be learned by any dog, and is always a crowd favorite! Dogs can be lifting their paws on cue within a few weeks, but the coordination of your routine can take longer. Your showy kicks will distract your audience from your subtle hand signals.

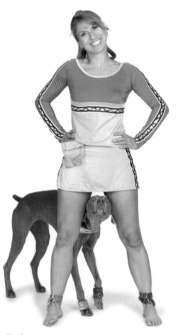
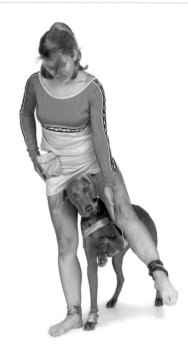
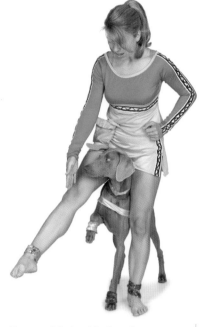

1 Start in a **peekaboo** position.

Reach your left hand down and forward as you say to "shake."

Use your right hand for "paw."

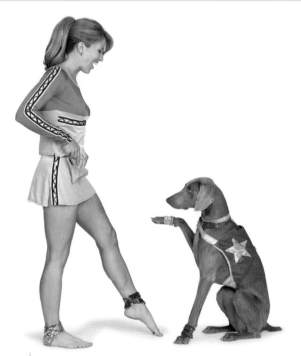
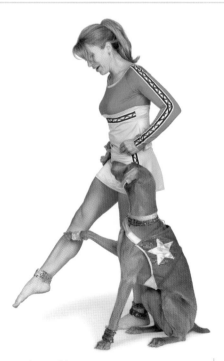

3 Try a variation with your dog facing you...

or at your side.

Chapter 11

The Thinking Man's Dog

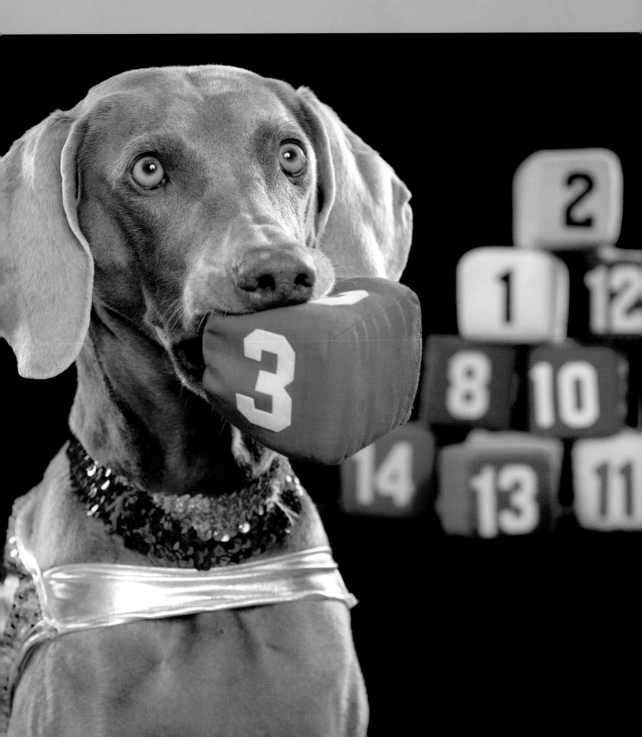

Intelligence

Intelligence in animals has always been a topic of debate, but any dog owner will tell you that they've been amazed by their dog's cleverness. As with humans, a dog's brainpower increases with use. The more you challenge your dog to use his comprehension, logic, and reasoning skills, the quicker he will grasp new concepts.

The tricks in this chapter have two things in common: they require a high level of thinking on your dog's part, and they are dependent on effective communication from you to your dog. Your dog is being asked not simply for a behavior, but a behavior based upon a communicated criteria. He needs to not just retrieve an object, but retrieve a specific one based upon a scent, hand signal, or verbal cue.

These difficult concepts can be mentally tiring for your dog. Use ten times more praise than negative feedback, as it is easy for your dog to become frustrated and discouraged. Even after he has learned the concept, he will occasionally make mistakes. Give him the benefit of the doubt as he is probably not picking out the wrong scent article or retrieving bumper on purpose. Learning is a lifelong process and these exercises will keep your dog mentally sharp throughout his years!

My Dog Can Count

TROUBLESHOOTING

DO HALF BARKS COUNT?
Your dog's barks need to be clear and countable. Use a crisp tone of voice when you tell him to "bark" and only reward a good result.

I GET ONE TOO MANY BARKS
For enthusiastic barkers, you may need to avert your eyes a second before that last bark to stop your dog in time.

BUILD ON IT! For a variation on this trick, ask your dog to count by tapping his paw instead of barking.

TIP! Communication is a two-way street. Make an effort to understand your dog's body language.

TEACH IT:

In this classic vaudeville schtick, your dog barks the correct number of times to solve a math problem. The believability of your dog's genius is dependent upon the subtlety of your signals. Your dog will start barking on cue and continue to bark until he receives another cue. You, I'm afraid, need to work out the math!

1 First, your dog needs to learn to bark multiple times. Signal your dog to **bark** (page 30) and continue to signal until you've elicited two barks. Maintain eye contact with your dog as he barks, and reward him after the second bark.

2 Your dog now needs to learn the signal to stop barking. This signal will eventually be the subtle aversion of your eyes. After your dog's second bark, lower your signaling hand, bow your head, avert your eyes, and say "stop." Reward your dog quickly if he stopped barking.

3 Increase the number of barks required and decrease dependence on your hand signal. You should be able to give the **bark** signal once, and have your dog continue to bark until you bow your head and break eye contact.

4 The rest is up to you! You can ask your dog a division problem, or have him bark once to answer "yes" and twice for "no." He can tell you his age (or your age if your audience has that much patience!)

VERBAL CUE
Bark, stop

HAND SIGNAL

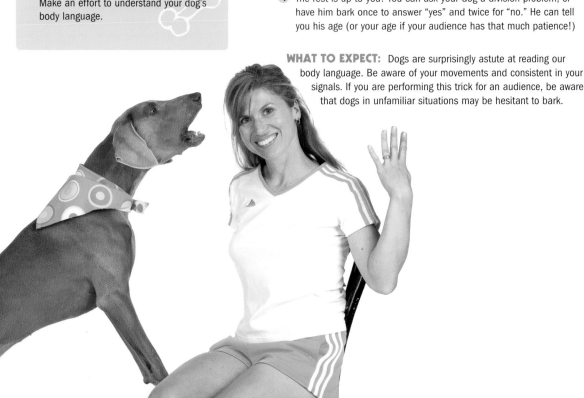

WHAT TO EXPECT: Dogs are surprisingly astute at reading our body language. Be aware of your movements and consistent in your signals. If you are performing this trick for an audience, be aware that dogs in unfamiliar situations may be hesitant to bark.

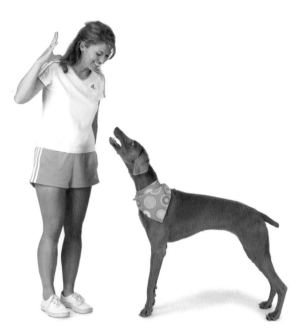

1 Signal your dog to **bark**, and reward after his second one.

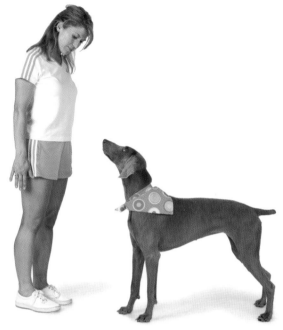

2 Lower your hand, head, and eyes and say "stop."

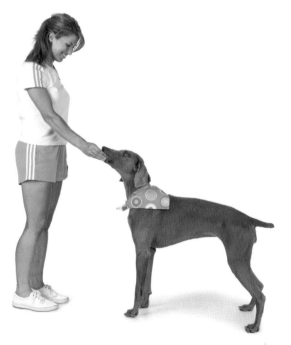

Reward your dog if he stopped barking.

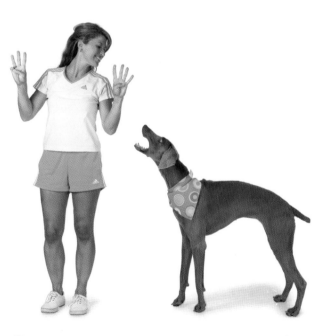

4 Ask your dog a math problem, and have him bark the answer!

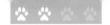
Discern Objects' Names

TROUBLESHOOTING

MY DOG IS SO EXCITED, HE GRABS THE FIRST OBJECT HE SEES
Hold your dog for ten seconds as you let the words sink in. Repeat your object name several times and let him focus on the object from afar.

BUILD ON IT! Rico, a border collie from Germany, demonstrated his knowledge of 200 object names!

TIP! Use objects names frequently with your dog. He can learn hundreds of words!

"Bumper, tennis ball, Kong, hike, dunk, treat ball, stick, toot, pink ringy, frisbee, dumbbell, bone-bone, squeak ... I have LOTS of toys!"

TEACH IT:

Your dog can learn to identify dozens of objects by name. Lay them all out on the floor and ask your dog to indicate a specific one.

VERBAL CUE
Find
[object name]

1. Start with a fun object whose name is already familiar to your dog, such as a bumper or tennis ball. Lay it in a clear area alongside two other nonenticing objects such as a hammer and hairbrush.

2. Point toward the objects and tell your dog to "find [bumper]." Praise him the moment he grabs the correct object. Use your **fetch** command (page 24) to encourage him to bring it to you. Reward him with a treat rather than by playing with the toy, as the latter would encourage him to only select toys from the pile of objects.

3. Add a second toy whose name is known to your dog. Alternate which one you tell him to find. If he chooses incorrectly, don't scold him, but rather don't acknowledge it one way or the other. Keep telling him to "find [object]."

WHAT TO EXPECT: This fun game really keeps your dog thinking. Practice with different toys and in different locations. Dogs learn the same way we do—by repetition—so keep practicing!

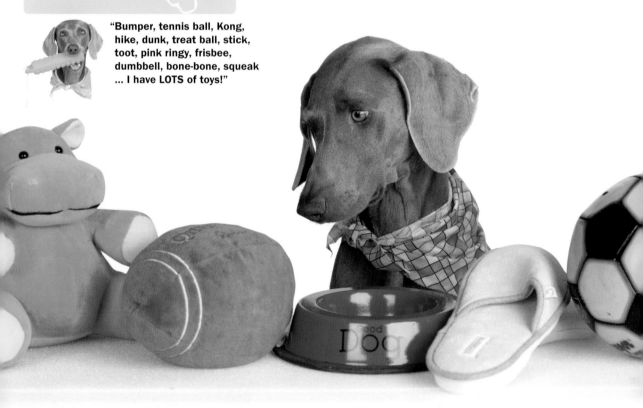

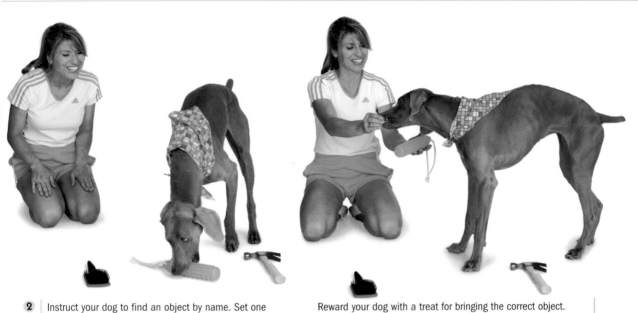

2 Instruct your dog to find an object by name. Set one
   familiar object amongst two unappealing objects.

Reward your dog with a treat for bringing the correct object.

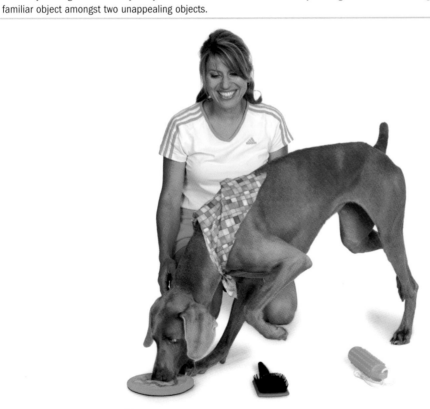

3 Add a second familiar object to the set. Alternate asking your dog to
   find each of the two familiar objects.

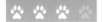
Directed Retrieve

TROUBLESHOOTING

MY DOG RETRIEVES THE OBJECT TO THE LEFT OF THE ONE INDICATED
Some dogs shy their head away from your hand, causing them to look left. Slip your hand through your dog's collar as you indicate the mark.

BUILD ON IT! Ready for the pros? Send your dog on a long-distance blind retrieve. If he veers off course, blow your whistle (to indicate him to look toward you and sit) and raise your right or left arm to indicate a new course of travel.

TIP! Spend at least twenty minutes every day training your dog.

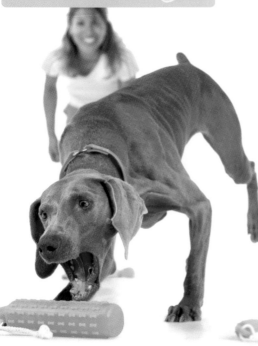

TEACH IT:

Your directional hand signal indicates to your dog the course of travel to find an object for retrieval. This exercise, using three white gloves, is part of the Utility Level Obedience test. A wagon wheel configuration of bumpers is used to test the abilities of a retrieving dog.

1 Set three plates about 15' (4.6 m) around you in a semicircle with a small treat placed on only one of the plates. With your dog sitting at your left and your toes pointed toward the plate with the treat, indicate to your dog the desired direction of travel—bend your knees slightly, open your hand, and run it from behind you straight toward the plate and alongside your dog's head while telling him "mark." Don't make eye contact with your dog, as you want him to look ahead to the plate rather than at you. Watch his head, and at the moment he is looking in the correct direction, send him with "get it!" This is a self-correcting training method, as your dog will only get the treat if he goes to the correct plate. If he veers in a wrong direction, do not let him finish the exercise, but call him back to your side. If your dog makes the same mistake twice in a row, move a few steps closer toward the correct plate.

VERBAL CUE
Mark
Get it!

HAND SIGNAL

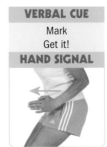

2 Now that your dog is reading your mark, replace the plates with three identical objects, such as white gloves or retrieving bumpers. This time your dog will be asked to **fetch** (page 24) the object. Remember to point your toes in the correct direction and send your dog only when his gaze is correctly directed.

3 Try a four-bumper wagon-wheel configuration—after a successful retrieve, toss the bumper back to its spot and select a new direction for the next retrieve. Try this configuration with eight or sixteen bumpers, or try a staggered configuration with bumpers at varying distances. Most difficult of all is a blind retrieve, where the bumpers are hidden in tall grass or behind a bush.

WHAT TO EXPECT: Sporting dogs generally have an easier time holding their mark (direction), while herding and toy breeds can have a harder time. The skill behind this exercise is your dog's ability to set out in a straight course in a designated direction. Once learned, this skill can have a variety of uses.

"My very very very favorite toy is Bumper. Bumper goes everywhere with me. I love Bumper. Bumper, Bumper, Bumper!"

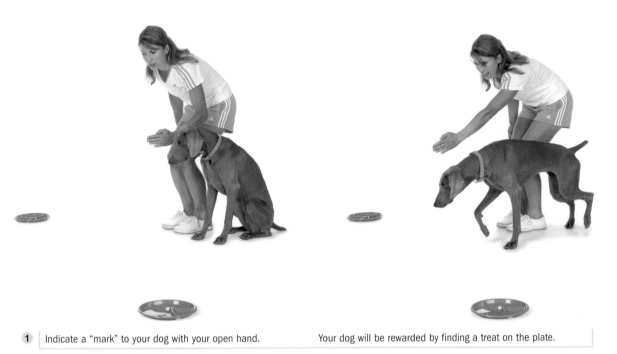

1 | Indicate a "mark" to your dog with your open hand. | Your dog will be rewarded by finding a treat on the plate.

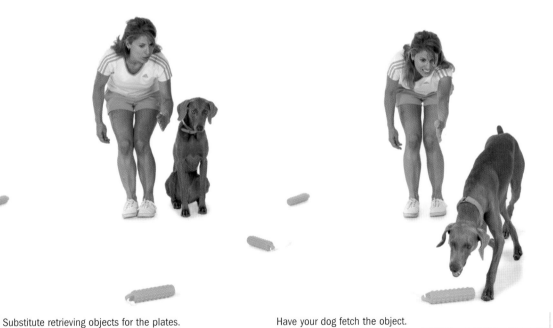

2 | Substitute retrieving objects for the plates. | Have your dog fetch the object.

Directed Jumping

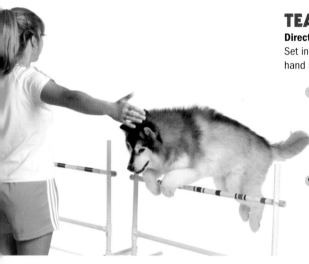

TEACH IT:

Directed jumping is one of the tests in sport of Utility Level Obedience. Set in front of two bar jumps, your dog jumps the one indicated by your hand signal.

1 Set your dog in a **stay** (page 18) directly in front of one of two side-by-side bar jumps. Position yourself on the other side of the jump and call your dog **over** (page 147). Repeat this exercise with the other jump.

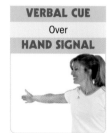

VERBAL CUE
Over
HAND SIGNAL

2 With your dog still positioned directly in front of one of the jumps, make it more difficult by standing centered between the two jumps. Signal your dog by raising the arm closest to the desired jump. In the beginning, you may wish to wave your arm or hold a treat bag or toy in your hand to focus your dog's attention in the correct direction.

3 Work incrementally until both you and your dog are centered between the jumps, facing each other. Use a verbal command and hand signal to indicate the desired jump.

WHAT TO EXPECT: Although this trick doesn't appear difficult to teach, there are often a variety of problems that crop up. This is a great exercise for building attention in your dog.

PREREQUISITES
Stay (page 18)
Jump over a bar (page 108)

TROUBLESHOOTING

MY DOG GOES AROUND THE JUMP
If your dog attempts to go around the jump, stop him before he gets all the way to you, and take him back to his starting position. Position yourself a little closer to the desired jump until he is successful.

BUILD ON IT! Starting with your dog at your side, send him to a **target** (page 145) past the jumps, and direct him to jump on his way back to you.

TIP! A slim, trim dog is a healthier dog—say no to table scraps and yes to exercise.

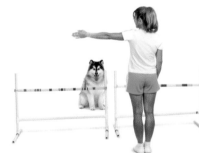

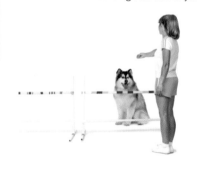

1 Set your dog directly in front of one of the jumps.

2 Stand centered between the jumps.

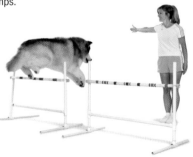

3 Finally, start with both you and your dog centered.

Pick a Card from a Deck

TEACH IT:

Your dog will learn to pull a single playing card from a fanned-out deck. Make your pooch a sensational part of your magic act!

1 Extend a single playing card toward your dog and tell him to "**take it**" (page 25). Hold it steady in your hand, without pushing it toward his mouth as the edges can be sharp.

VERBAL CUE
Take it

2 Now hold three cards in a wide fan as you instruct your dog to take one. Reward him for any card he takes.

3 When you are ready to add a fourth card, extend one card in front of the others so your dog can take it easier. As your dog improves, extend it less and less until it is even with the other cards. If your dog is pulling out more than one card at a time, coax him to be gentle by slowly saying "easy." If two cards are pulled out, say "whoops!" and try again without rewarding.

4 Are you ready to try an entire deck? Fan the cards as wide as you can and extend several slightly beyond the others.

WHAT TO EXPECT: Small dogs tend to learn this trick easier, but any dog can be picking a card within a week. Keep refining his skills until he does it like a pro. Don't be surprised if you come home early to find a dog poker game in your living room!

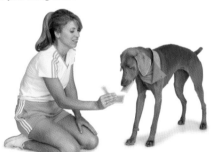

2 Hold three cards in a wide fan.

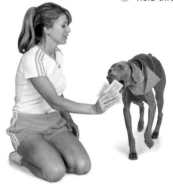

3 Extend on card above the others.

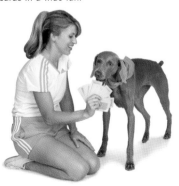

4 Fan the whole deck, staggering some.

PREREQUISITES
Take it (page 24)

TROUBLESHOOTING

MY DOG TAKES THE TINIEST EDGE OF THE CARD
Your dog should take the card firmly so as not to risk dropping it. Give some resistance as he pulls a card, causing him to grip harder.

BUILD ON IT! Your dog will be a magician with the help of a "stripper deck," which has a slightly tapered side. If a card is removed and inserted back into the deck in the other direction, it will be the only card tapered in the opposite direction.

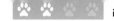
Food Refusal

"What's an oxymoron?"

TEACH IT:

In this this trick, your dog turns his head away from food offered from your hand. Add humor to this trick by explaining "my dog only eats *kosher* hot dogs," or asking "what do you think of my home cooking?"

1   Facing your dog, extend a treat toward him.

2   When he shows interest in the treat, tell him "yuck" in a disapproving tone and pull your hand away or lightly bop him on the nose.

VERBAL CUE

Yuck

3   Repeat this process until your dog looks away from your hand. Watch closely, and mark this instant by saying "good!" Release him from this exercise with your release word "OK" and give him the treat.

4   Accept small aversions of his eyes at the beginning and gradually require him to turn away for longer periods of time. Once he has the hang of it, use your release word to signify that he may now take the treat from your hand. "My mistake, it *is* a kosher hot dog!"

WHAT TO EXPECT: Most dogs can learn this trick within a few weeks. Dogs are prone to cheating, so be consistent with your criteria for success. You can move your hand from left to his right, and require him to change his head position to continue to look away from the treat.

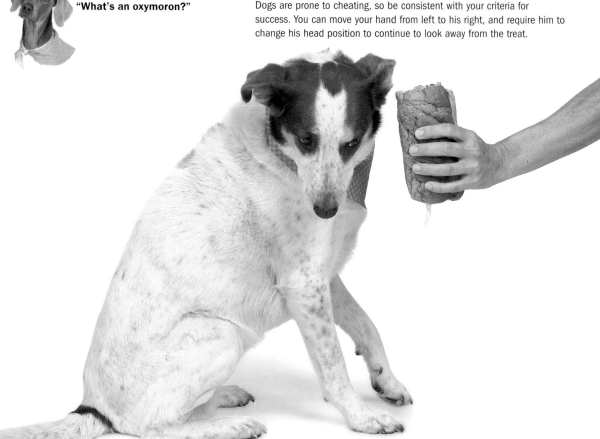

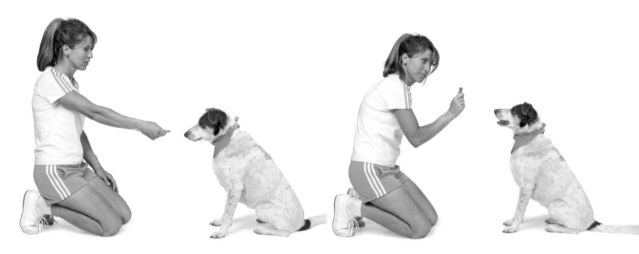

1 Extend a treat toward your dog.

2 When he shows interest, pull your hand away.

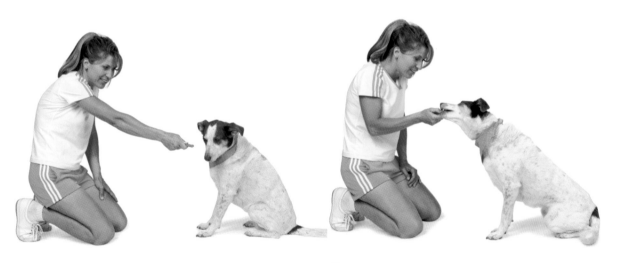

3 Watch closely for the moment your dog looks away.

4 Use your release word to signify that he may now take the treat.

Find the Object with My Scent

TROUBLESHOOTING

MY DOG IS SUDDENLY HAVING TROUBLE
Have you changed your soap, hand lotion, or laundry detergent? How about your diet or medication that may affect your scent? Was someone smoking near your articles? New flea spray? Carpets cleaned? Visitor at the house? Changes in scent can temporarily confuse your dog.

BUILD ON IT! Continue scent training with **track a person's scent trail** (page 194).

TEACH IT:

Utility Obedience competition requires your dog to search twelve identical objects and retrieve the one with your scent. Leather and metal dumbbells are commonly used for this exercise, but wooden dowels, metal jar lids, or even clean silverware can be used.

1 It is vital to this exercise that the articles used are free of your scent. Air them out for several days between uses and handle them using tongs. Mark them with unique numbers so you can tell which is the scented one!

VERBAL CUE
Find mine

2 Using pegboard or a mat with holes poked through, tie down two out of three identical articles. Scent the third by rubbing it in your palms for ten seconds, and also with a little of the treat you are using. Place the scented article with the other two, and instruct your dog to **fetch** (page 24). Be very gentle when training scent work. Avoid saying "no," but instead let your dog figure out on his own that only one article is retrievable and not tied down. Praise him the second he takes the correct article in his mouth, and reward him for bringing it to you.

3 Tie additional unscented articles to the mat. If your dog has trouble finding the free one, encourage him to keep looking. Phase out the scent of the treat, and use only your scent on the object.

4 Now try it with all the objects not tied down. If your dog picks up a wrong one, just ignore it as he may change his mind on his own. If he starts to bring an incorrect article back to you, use an encouraging tone to tell him to keep looking. Do not accept the wrong item.

WHAT TO EXPECT: Scent work is one of the most difficult exercises to train, and dogs can be particularly sensitive to criticism in this area. If your dog feels he has been reprimanded for choosing an incorrect article, he may doubt his understanding of your wishes and use an avoidance technique to get out of doing the exercise.

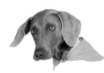

"Things I don't like: fire ants, waiting in line, pineapple."

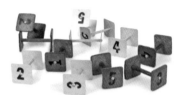

1 The articles should be free from your scent and marked for identification.

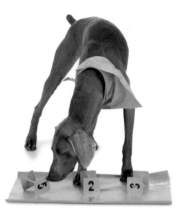

2 Tie down two out of three articles. Scent the third, and place it alongside the others.

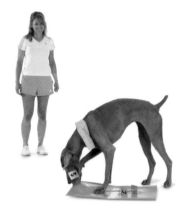

Your dog will not be able to retrieve the unscented articles.

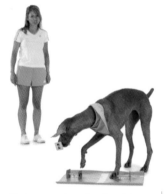

Praise your dog when he picks up the scented article.

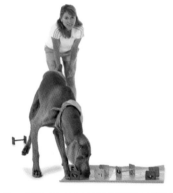

3 Tie additional unscented articles to the mat.

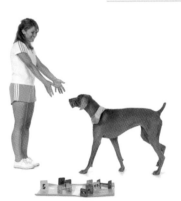

4 Have all the articles not tied down.

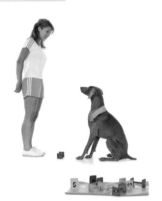

Do not accept a wrong article from your dog.

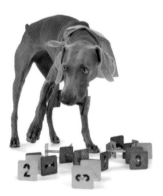

Encourage your dog, and soon he'll be sniffing out your article reliably!

Contraband Search

TROUBLESHOOTING

WHAT KIND OF TEA SHOULD I USE?
Many dogs are crazy about mint!

CAN MY DOG FIND A TEA BAG IN SOMEONE'S POCKET?
Yes, but it will be more difficult, as the scent will be confined to a smaller area. The longer the tea bag sits in their pocket however, the easier its scent will be to detect.

BUILD ON IT! Now that your dog is familiar with scent work, try **find the object with my scent** (page 190).

TIP! To perform confidently and happily, your dog must have a clear idea of expectations.

TEACH IT:

Similar to a drug-detection dog, your K-9 will sniff out contraband. Three volunteers participate, one of whom is given a tea bag. Your dog searches for the "contraband" tea bag scent, and indicates the possessor. Train your dog to indicate the find with a signal such as sitting, lying down, or nuzzling the tea bag.

VERBAL CUE
Scent
Find it

HAND SIGNAL

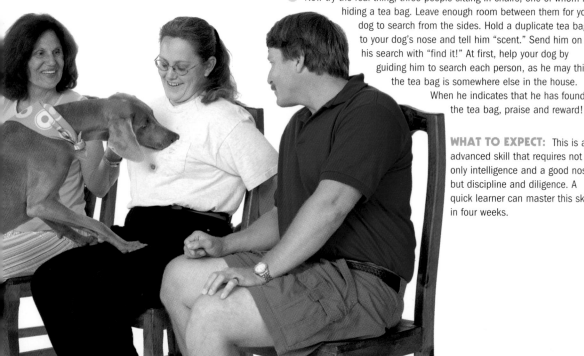

1 Build on your dog's knowledge of **finding hidden treats** (page 98), by transitioning to finding a tea bag. Hold the tea bag to your dog's nose, and use the word "scent" to indicate this is the scent to seek.

2 Hide the tea bag in an obvious spot, and place a treat on top of it. Instruct your dog to "find it" and let him eat the treat when he does.

3 After several repetitions, rub the treat on the tea bag, and hide the tea bag only. Encourage your dog as he searches, even pointing and running alongside him. He will probably come close to the tea bag, but not know what to do. At this point, place a treat on top of the tea bag, and praise him when he gets it. This transition period will be a little confusing, as your dog learns that he is searching for the tea bag, and not the treat. Eventually, you will hide the tea bag only, and when your dog finds it you can toss him a treat.

4 Once your dog has the hang of searching out the tea bag in hidden spots, try placing in on a person's knee, as they sit on the floor.

5 Now try the real thing; three people sitting in chairs, one of whom is hiding a tea bag. Leave enough room between them for your dog to search from the sides. Hold a duplicate tea bag to your dog's nose and tell him "scent." Send him on his search with "find it!" At first, help your dog by guiding him to search each person, as he may think the tea bag is somewhere else in the house. When he indicates that he has found the tea bag, praise and reward!

WHAT TO EXPECT: This is an advanced skill that requires not only intelligence and a good nose, but discipline and diligence. A quick learner can master this skill in four weeks.

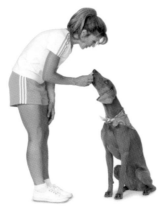

1 Hold a tea bag to your dog's nose as you tell him "scent."

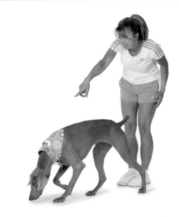

2 Place a treat on top of the tea bag and have your dog "find it."

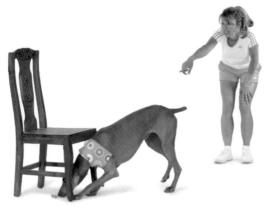

3 Rub a treat on the tea bag and reward your dog when he finds it.

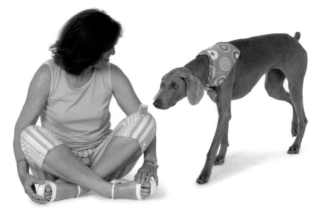

4 Place the tea bag on a person's knee.

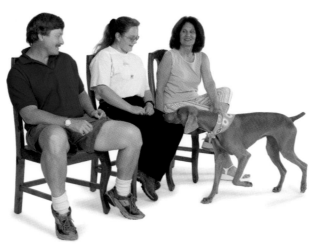

5 Have your dog search several people for the "contraband" tea bag.

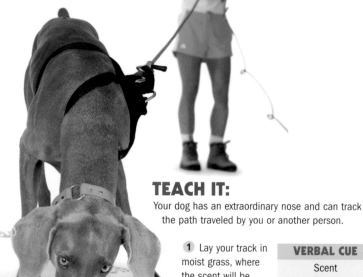
Track a Person's Scent Trail

PREREQUISITES
Down (page 16)
Helpful: Easter egg hunt (page 98

TROUBLESHOOTING

MY DOG STAYS CLOSE TO MY LEGS INSTEAD OF LEADING
Keep your lips zipped and let his instinct take over. The more you talk to your dog, the more he will look to you for direction.

I'M BUNDLED UP FOR COLD WEATHER— AM I LEAVING ENOUGH SCENT?
Yes, your scent will come through your clothes. Your dog can also smell the scent of the smashed grass blades under your feet.

BUILD ON IT! Expert trackers can follow aged tracks with several turns and over a variety of surfaces.

TIP! A dog's sniffing behavior involves taking short, deep inhalations that pass air over olfactory receptors deep in the dog's snout.

"Track a person? I thought I was tracking hot dogs!"

TEACH IT:
Your dog has an extraordinary nose and can track the path traveled by you or another person.

1 Lay your track in moist grass, where the scent will be easiest to detect.

VERBAL CUE
Scent
Track

Scuff your feet at the beginning of your track to create a "scent pad," and continue scuffing as you walk about 50 yards (46 m) in a straight line. Drop odoriferous treats, such as hot dog slices, along your path every few yards and use small cones or flags to remind yourself of your path. Leave an object with your scent, such as a sock, at the end of the track. Stuff some treats inside the sock to capture your dog's interest.

2 Outfit your dog in a harnesses and 12' (3.7 m) lead and bring him to the scent pad. Tell him to "track" and let him find the first treat left along your trail. Unlike in obedience, when tracking your dog leads— showing *you* where to go. Walk slowly, allowing him to pull forward. Do not reprimand him for veering off track, but do not let him pull you off course.

3 When a working tracking dog finds a scented object, he is trained to signal the handler by lying down. When your dog gets to the end of your track and nuzzles the sock, tell him to lie **down** (page 16) and reward him with a treat from inside.

4 Now try a gradual 90-degree turn in your track. Note that your track holds its scent for a day or more, so use a variety of training locations. Take note of the wind direction. If your dog is traveling downwind from your track, it may be that he is airscenting. Graduate to a 20' (6.1 m) lead and farther spaced treats as your dog becomes more independent. Increase difficulty by aging the tracks before following them.

WHAT TO EXPECT: It is often hard to distinguish between a dog off-track and a dog picking up scent that has blown downwind. Have trust that your dog knows his job and assume your role as coach rather than teacher. Dogs enjoy scent work and can be tracking a trail of hot dogs within a few weeks.

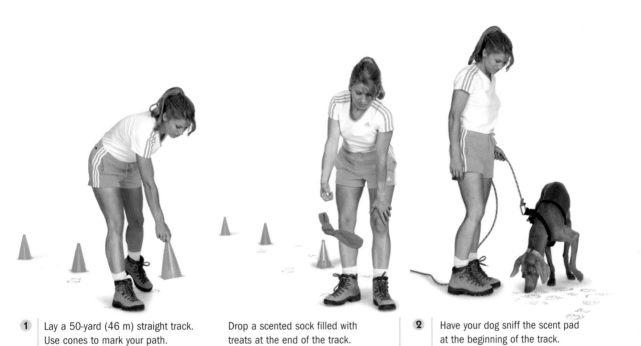

1 Lay a 50-yard (46 m) straight track. Use cones to mark your path.

Drop a scented sock filled with treats at the end of the track.

2 Have your dog sniff the scent pad at the beginning of the track.

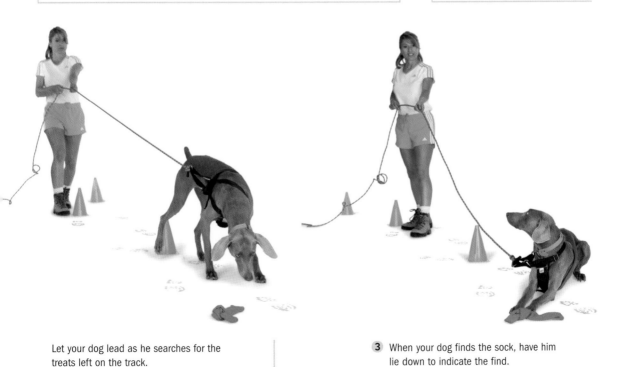

Let your dog lead as he searches for the treats left on the track.

3 When your dog finds the sock, have him lie down to indicate the find.

Chapter 12
Love Me, Love My Dog

Puppy dog eyes can melt the hardest of hearts and unravel the strongest of wills because we, after all, love our dogs. Obedience trainers and dog behaviorists may scorn as we sleep with furry foot warmers or perch our pooch on our lap and (heaven forbid!) kiss him on the lips. But rules are made to be broken, and we promise … we won't tell!

"Quo me amat, amat et canem meam." Love me, love my dog. This Latin proverb quoted to Saint Bernard has been repeated in almost every language throughout the centuries.

Go ahead and celebrate the close bond between you and your dog with the intimate tricks in this chapter. These expressive behaviors will endear him to all!

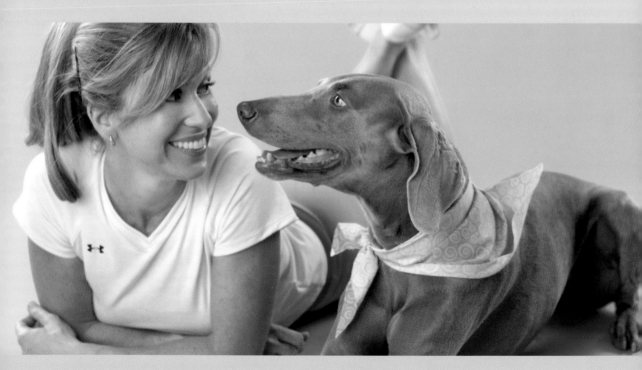

Kisses

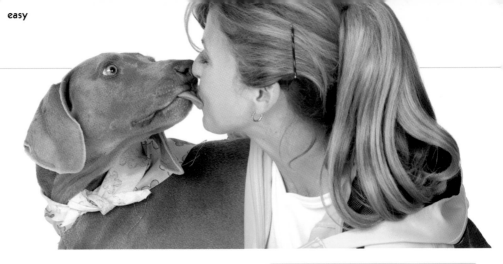

TEACH IT:

Your dog licks or noses the lips or cheek of you or another person.

1 Sit at "doggy-level." Give the verbal cue and place a treat between your teeth as you lean forward. Allow your dog to take the treat, and praise him with "good kisses!"

2 If you do not wish your dog to kiss you on your lips (although I can't imagine why!), put some peanut butter on your cheek, point to it while saying "kisses," and let him lick it off.

3 With a treat held behind your back, point to your lips or cheek and tell your dog "kisses!" When he licks or noses you, mark the instant with "good!" and reward him with the treat.

4 Now try it with someone else. Have a helper apply some peanut butter to their cheek. Point to it and cue your dog. When he licks your helper's cheek, tell him "good," and reward him. Step back and send your dog a farther distance to give kisses. Phase out the peanut butter and have your dog return to you for his treat.

WHAT TO EXPECT: Dogs will often learn this trick within a week, although shy dogs may require more coaxing.

| VERBAL CUE |
| Kisses |
| HAND SIGNAL |

TROUBLESHOOTING

MY DOG BITES MY LIP
Address this issue separately by telling your dog "easy" as you allow him to take treats. Bop him on the nose if he bites, and say "ouch!"

MY DOG IS SCARED NEAR MY FACE
Your dog is putting himself in a submissive position by coming close to your mouth (which in dog culture could lead to a bite). This trick requires trust. Try holding the treat several inches from your mouth, and as he reaches for it, bring it closer to your face.

TIP! In dog packs, a dog will lick the lips of a more dominant dog, as a way of showing subservience

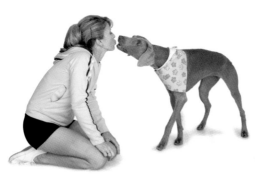

1 Let your dog to take a treat from your teeth.

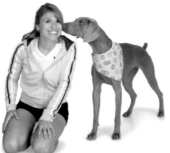

2 Put peanut butter on your cheek.

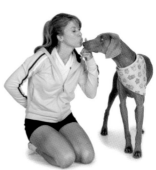

3 Point to your lips for a kiss.

Paws on My Arm

TEACH IT:

If your pet peeve is a pet that jumps on guests, teach him to welcome visitors with **paws on their arm** to give him a safe and manageable way to show his enthusiasm.

1 Sit on the floor with your dog on your left. Raise your left arm in front of him and lure his head upward with a treat in your right hand. Your dog will probably place one or both paws on your forearm, in an effort to reach the treat, but if he doesn't you can coax his paws onto your arm with your hands. Once your dog is in the correct position, with his paws resting on your arm, allow him to nibble treats from your hand.

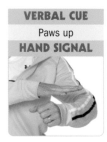

| VERBAL CUE |
| Paws up |
| HAND SIGNAL |

2 Try this exercise while standing up. Use the verbal cue and hand signal. You may wish to hold the treat in your mouth until you are ready to give it to your dog to keep him from becoming distracted by it (hot dogs or cheese work well).

WHAT TO EXPECT: Dog's can often learn this trick within a few training sessions. Your guests are sure to thank you!

TROUBLESHOOTING

MY DOG PUTS ONLY ONE PAW ON MY ARM

To start, you may have to use your hand to guide his second paw up.

MY DOG IS STILL JUMPING ON PEOPLE!

This hand signal will become an invitation for your dog to raise himself to your arm. Be clear with your rules—without an invitation, your dog should be reprimanded for jumping on people (assuming that is your rule).

BUILD ON IT! Once you've mastered **paws on my arm**, use a similar action to learn **say your prayers** (page 42)!

TIP! Position your arm perpendicular to your body and have your dog approach from the outside so as to prevent him from knocking you over or overextending your shoulder.

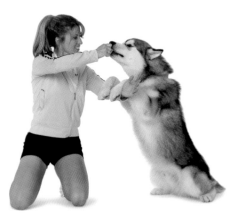

1 Lure your dog onto your arm and allow him to nibble a treat.

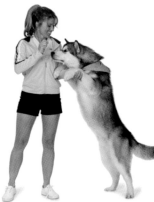

2 Repeat this exercise while standing.

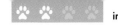
Head Down

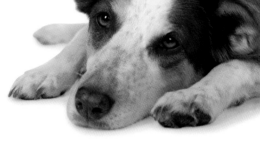

TEACH IT:

From a down position, your dog lowers his head to rest upon the floor. This is a common trick for movie dogs. "Aww, the doggy looks sad!"

1. Kneel to the side of your dog as he rests in a down position. Hold a treat on the floor, out of reach in front of him. Cue "head down" while using your other hand to gently push his head to the floor using pressure points behind his ears.

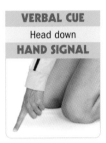

VERBAL CUE
Head down
HAND SIGNAL

2. Hold him for a few seconds with his chin resting on the floor between his paws, then praise and slide your treat toward him. Allow him to take the treat and then give your release word "OK" and release his head so he can chew. If your dog is very resistant to your physical manipulation, reward the instant his chin touches the floor, so as not to cause him to struggle.

3. Gradually lighten your touch on his head, so that you do short taps rather than constant pressure. Once his head is down, instruct him to "stay" a few seconds before rewarding. Always present your reward on the floor, so your dog isn't tempted to look up for it.

WHAT TO EXPECT: In its final stage, you should be able to stand some distance from your dog and point on the ground while giving the verbal cue. Submissive dogs will have an easier time with this behavior than dominant dogs. Train calmly and gently, and gauge your dog's anxiety level so as not to push him past his comfort zone.

TROUBLESHOOTING

MY DOG RUNS AWAY WHEN I TRY TO TRAIN THIS TRICK

Physically manipulating your dog is a slippery slope. He may think you are dominating him or punishing him by pushing his head down. Progress slowly and gently with this trick, and only practice two or three times per session. Praise lavishly!

BUILD ON IT! Lift your pointed finger up from the floor to teach "head up."

TIP! Old dogs want to make you proud as well! Ask them for a behavior they can achieve, and praise lavishly!

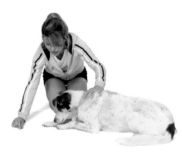

1. A combination of a food lure and your hand pressure will guide your dog's head down.

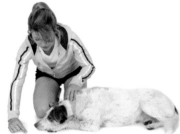

2. Slide the treat to your dog while keeping him in the proper position.

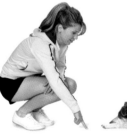
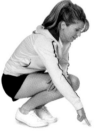

3. Use your hand signal to focus your dog's attention downward.

Cover Your Eyes

TEACH IT:

Your dog hides his eyes by hooking his paw over his muzzle.

1. Stick a sticky note or piece of tape to your dog's muzzle and encourage him to "cover, get it!" One swipe at his face should be enough to dislodge the paper. Praise him with "good cover!"

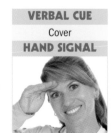

VERBAL CUE
Cover
HAND SIGNAL

2. With your dog laying down, stick the note to the center of his head, just above his eyes. He will have a harder time swatting at this spot and will eventually poke his head under one wrist. Perfect! Be ready to reward him in the spot where his head pokes under his paw.

3. Alternate between using the sticky note and just tapping his head in the spot where you normally stick the sticky note. Use "stay" to get your dog to hold the position for a few seconds.

4. Try it from a sitting position. Place the sticky note on the bridge of your dog's nose and when he raises his paw to swat at it, reward him under his arm. As you wean off the sticky note, he may try to get away with merely waving, without touching his face. In this case, go back to using a sticky note. Eventually, stand up while giving the cue to encourage your dog's head higher. Try it with your dog in different positions: sit, down, or bow.

WHAT TO EXPECT: This method of training is so natural that your dog should be swiping the note right away. After about a month, or 200 repetitions, your dog should have the hang of an eye cover with the aid of the sticky note. It could take a lot longer, however, until he has it mastered without that aid.

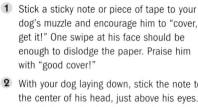

TROUBLESHOOTING

MY DOG SHAKES HIS HEAD INSTEAD OF PAWING AT THE STICKY NOTE

Use a stronger adhesive tape so your dog can't merely shake it off. Cue him to **shake hands** (page 22) to give him the idea to use his paw. Stick the note in different places: above or below his eye or on top of his head.

MY DOG JUST SITS THERE WITH THE PAPER STUCK TO HIS NOSE!

Your dignified dog needs to be encouraged to attack the object, as he would a bug on his nose. Touch the paper to make him aware of it and use your voice to excite him.

TIP! Take your dog on a trip or errand. It will be good for his social skills and he'll enjoy the change of scenery.

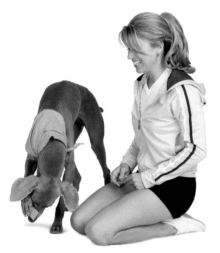

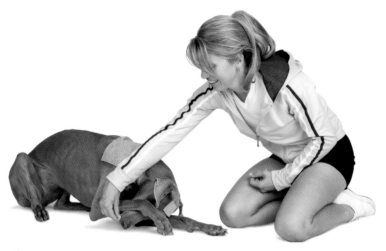

1. Encourage your dog to swipe at a sticky note on his face.

2. While laying down, your dog will poke his head under his paw.

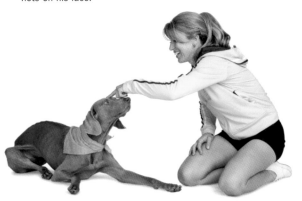

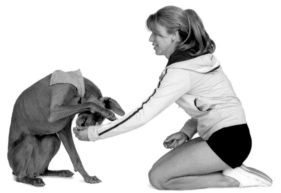

3. Just tap the spot on his head instead of using a sticky note.

4. Go back to using the sticky note, but this time in the sitting position.

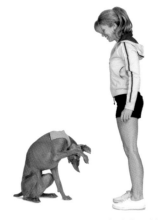

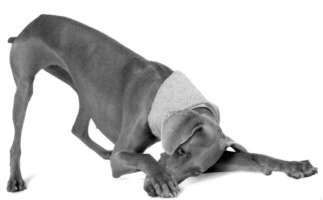

Stand up to encourage your dog's head higher.

Try an eye cover in a bow position.

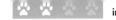

Wave Good-bye

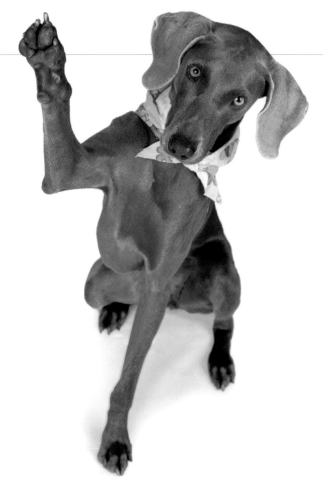

PREREQUISITES
Shake hands (page 22)

TROUBLESHOOTING

AS I MOVE AWAY FROM MY DOG, HE KEEPS MOVING TOWARD ME, TRYING TO TOUCH MY HAND

Stand a few feet away from your dog with your hand outstretched toward him as you cue him. At the last second, pull your hand away so that he is pawing the air. Reward this!

MY DOG STANDS UP

Put him back in a sit before continuing to train. He will have higher extension from a sitting position.

BUILD ON IT! Sit alongside your dog as you both **wave good-bye** together.

TIP! Sometimes, your dog offers an unexpected, but cute, behavior. Don't miss that opportunity! Reward it and try to elicit it again.

TEACH IT:
Your dog waves his paw high in the air.

1. With your dog sitting, face him and have him **shake hands** (page 22).

2. Say "shake, bye-bye" and extend your hand a little higher than you normally would to shake hands. Your dog won't be able to hold his paw that high, so his motion will look like he is pawing at your hand.

3. Draw your hand slightly away from your dog, so he can just barely reach your fingers.

4. Pull your hand back at the last second so he is not touching it at all, but merely pawing the air. Be sure to praise him, so he understands that the desired behavior is the waving motion, as opposed to the actual touch.

WHAT TO EXPECT: With a solid shake, your dog can transition to a wave within a few training sessions.

VERBAL CUE
Bye bye
HAND SIGNAL

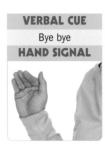

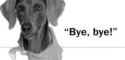

"Bye, bye!"

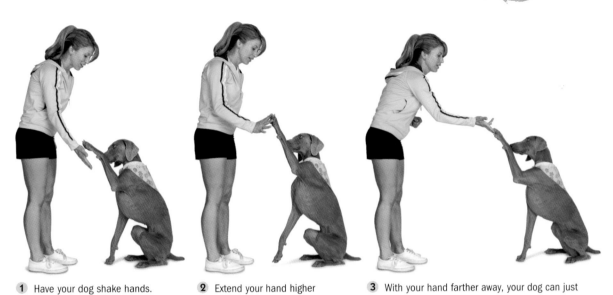

1 Have your dog shake hands.

2 Extend your hand higher than normal.

3 With your hand farther away, your dog can just barely reach your fingers.

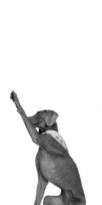

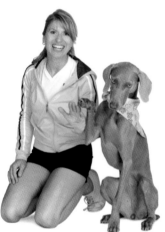

4 Pull your hand back at the last second so your dog paws the air.

Transition to the hand signal.

"Bye, bye!"

APPENDIX A: TRICKS BY SKILL LEVEL

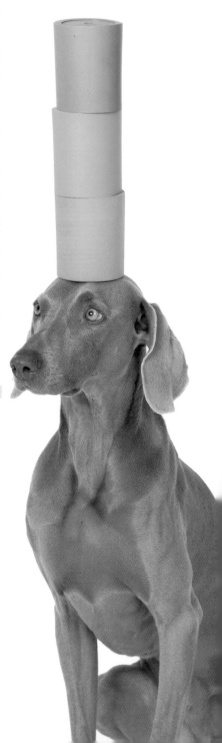

EASY

INTERMEDIATE

ADVANCED

EXPERT

APPENDIX B: TRICKS BY SPORT

AGILITY

hoop jump	125
jump over a bar	108
teeter-totter	148
touch a target	145
tunnel	143
under/over	146
weave poles	150

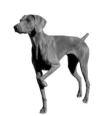

DISC DOG

beginning disc dog	120
disc vault off my leg	122
jump into my arms	112
jump over my back	110
jump over my knee	109
jump through my arms	126
summersault/handstand vault	114

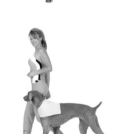

DOG DANCING/FREESTYLE

back up	161
chorus line kicks	176
figure 8's	172
head down	199
heel forward and backward	160
jump for joy	175
jump through my arms	126
leg weave	170
moonwalk	174
paws on my arm	198
peekaboo!	52
place (circle to my left side)	166
rollover	31
side (swing to my left side)	168
sit pretty/beg	28
spin circles	162
take a bow	164
wave good-bye	202

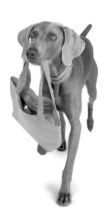

HELPER DOG/SERVICE DOG

bring me a beer from the fridge	74
bring me a tissue	82
carry my purse	44
discern objects names	182
fetch my slippers	36
find the remote/car keys	78
get the phone when it rings	67
get your leash	37
kennel up	43
mail carrier	76
newspaper delivery	40
open/close a door	70
pull on a rope	73
push a shopping cart	80
ring a bell to come inside	72

tidy up your toys	46
turn off the light	68

HUNTING/RETRIEVING

directed retrieve	184
dog on point	104
drop it/give	26
fetch/take it	24

OBEDIENCE

come	19
directed jumping	186
directed retrieve	184
doggy push-ups	54
down	16
drop it/give	26
fetch/take it	24
find the object with my scent	190
heel forward and backward	160
jump over a bar	108
place (circle to my left side)	166
side (swing to my left side)	168
sit	15
stay	18

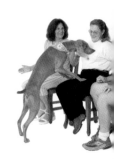

SEARCH AND RESCUE/POLICE DOG

climb a ladder	152
contraband search	192
crawl	144
easter egg hunt	98
food refusal	188
hide and seek	94
roll a barrel	154
track a person's scent trail	194

THERAPY DOG

cover your eyes	200
head down	199
kisses	197
paws on my arm	198
say your prayers	42
shake hands—left and right	22
speak	30

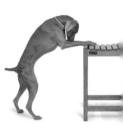

TRACKING

find the object with my scent	190
hide and seek	94
track a person's scent trail	194

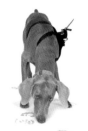

ABOUT THE AUTHORS

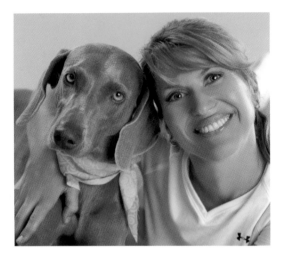

Five year old Weimaraner, **Chalcy**, is the most recognized dog in the country. She and her owner and trainer, **Kyra Sundance**, have entertained audiences worldwide with their trick dog show, performing at fairs, circuses, schools, and sporting event halftime shows. Audiences have been amazed by television performances on the *Ellen DeGeneres Show, Entertainment Tonight, Best Damn Sports Show Period,* and the *Tonight Show* where Jay Leno deemed Chalcy "World's Smartest Dog!" Complex routines, comic antics, and obvious love for each other are an inspiration to animal enthusiasts.

In addition to tricks, Kyra and Chalcy spent years achieving expert ranking in the competitive dog sport of obedience, agility, jumping, hunting, retrieving, and versatility.

Kyra's step-by-step approach to dog trick training has benefited hundreds of students as they rediscovered the joys of their dog. Kyra utilizes positive training methods that emphasize bonding, collaboration, reward, and instinctive dog communication styles.

Kyra and Chalcy live with Kyra's husband, Randy Banis, on a ranch in California's Mojave Desert.

ABOUT THE PHOTOGRAPHER

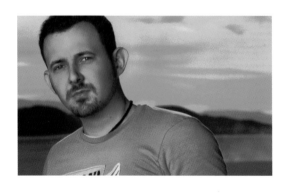

Born in Baltimore, Maryland, **Nick Saglimbeni** moved to Los Angeles in 1997 to pursue cinematography at the top-ranked USC School of Cinema. After shooting several commercials, music videos, and short films, Nick was recognized in 2003 by the American Society of Cinematographers with a Heritage Award. That same year, after hearing countless stories from frustrated actors and models who were unable to find good photographers, Nick opened SlickforceStudio, a cutting-edge photo studio in downtown LA. Clients immediately responded to the cinematic nature of Nick's work, and the studio quickly gained international recognition. Nick's work has been featured in many major magazines, and he continues to shoot for film and television. You can see more of his work at www.slickforce.com.

ACKNOWLEDGMENTS

Thanks to Heidi Horn (production assistant, bandanna co-ordinator, dog petter, and Kyra's mother) and Claire Doré (assistant trainer, consultant, and dog motivator), and especially to all the beautiful, talented, and hard-working dogs: Dana (Aussie mix), Kwest & Kwin (Alaskan malamutes), Sutton (yellow Lab), Gina (rough collie), Skippy (parson russell mix), Cricket (Chihuahua), and Chalcy (Weimaraner).

IN MEMORIAM

A short time before this book went to press, Dana's life was tragically taken when she was hit by a car and killed instantly. Dana (below, far right) had an esteemed career as an animal actor, where she performed for film and television as well as live shows. She was an extremely intelligent dog with a kind and gentle soul. She will be missed by all those who knew and loved her, and especially by her owner, Claire.

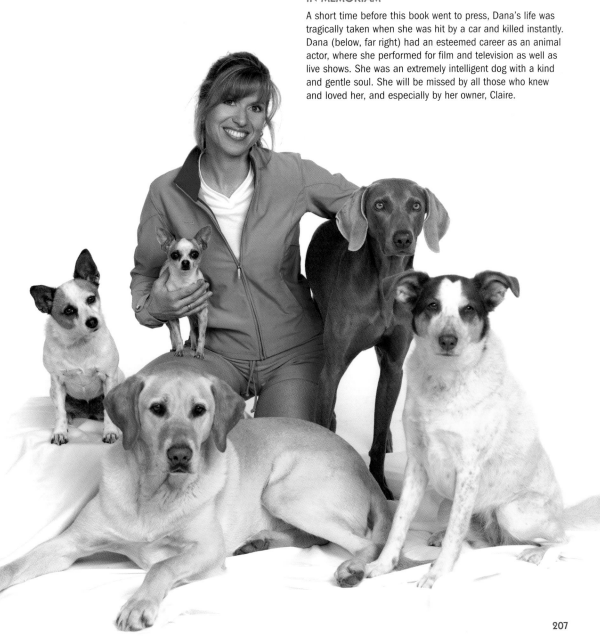

50 MORE TRICKS!

1   ABCs identification
2   Baseball
3   Breakdance: rub your back on the floor
4   Chase your tail
5   Cock your head to one side
6   Cross your paws
7   Dangling rope: use mouth and paw to pull up
8   Deposit coin into piggy bank
9   Dig
10   Drink from a fountain
11   Find a lost object
12   Guard an object
13   Growl/bare teeth
14   Hi-ho silver away/rear on hind legs
15   Jump into the car
16   Lead a person by the wrist
17   Lick lips/act hungry
18   Nod in agreement
19   Nose touch to hand
20   Object placement
21   Paws up
22   Pony ride: stand on my back as I crawl
23   Pull on harness/pull a cart
24   Push things with paw (doors, drawers)
25   Ring around the rosy
26   Ring bell by pulling string
27   Ring bell with nose
28   Ring bell with paw
29   Roll over with ball between front paws
30   Rub muzzle on floor
31   Scratch yourself
32   Shake an object
33   Shake head in disagreement
34   Shake yourself
35   Sing
36   Skateboard
37   Sneeze
38   Soft mouth: carry a raw egg
39   Spin with front paws on a stool
40   Stop at the curb
41   Stop at the front door
42   Stop dead on cue
43   Swim
44   Take money and bring it to you!
45   Tap your paw to count
46   Toss a toy in the air
47   Volleyball with a balloon
48   Walk backward up stairs
49   Walk on forequarters
50   Yawn

This page was supposed to be called the "conclusion." But this is not the conclusion to your dog training at all, but rather the first steps in a lifelong endeavor. Now that you have some skills under your belt and ideas and guidance for training, your adventure is just beginning!

As you've read through the tricks in this book, you've probably noticed similarities in training techniques—give a cue, lure your dog into position, give the reward, up the ante. As you get ready to train new tricks, original tricks, tricks that are unique to you and your dog, use the strategies you've learned to figure out the methods.

Test your training creativity by running down the list to the left, and thinking about how you would train these tricks. How would you get your dog to lick his lips (number 17 in the list)? Why, you put peanut butter on his nose, of course! How about to use a soft mouth to carry an egg (number 38)? Train with a stick wrapped in wire, which would hurt his teeth if he bared down. Cross your paws (number 6)? Have your dog do a paw shake while in a down position. Gradually move your hand to the side, until his shake crosses over his other paw. Sing (number 35)? When does your dog normally howl? At a siren or other noise? Most dogs will sing to a harmonica if you hit the right note. I'm sure you get the idea.

Our dog's lives are far too short, and the time we have to enjoy with them passes quickly. Make the most of it!

www.101dogtricks.com

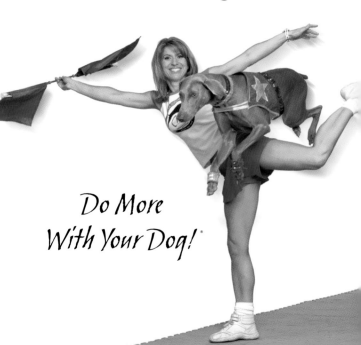

Do More With Your Dog!